T0271474

Step-by-Step Help for Children with ADHD

Step-by-Step Help for
CHILDREN
with ADHD

A Guide for Parents
SECOND EDITION

**Cathy Laver-Bradbury,
Margaret Thompson, Anne Weeks,
David Daley** and **Edmund Sonuga-Barke**

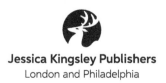

Jessica Kingsley Publishers
London and Philadelphia

First published in Great Britain in 2025 by Jessica Kingsley Publishers
An imprint of John Murray Press

1

A CIP catalogue record for this title is available from the
British Library and the Library of Congress

ISBN 978 1 80501 107 1
eISBN 978 1 80501 108 8

Printed and bound in Great Britain by TJ Books Ltd

Jessica Kingsley Publishers' policy is to use papers that are natural,
renewable and recyclable products and made from wood grown in sus-
tainable forests. The logging and manufacturing processes are expected
to conform to the environmental regulations of the country of origin.

Jessica Kingsley Publishers
Carmelite House
50 Victoria Embankment
London EC4Y 0DZ

www.jkp.com

John Murray Press
Part of Hodder & Stoughton Ltd
An Hachette Company

The authorised representative in the EEA is Hachette Ireland, 8 Castlecourt Centre,
Castleknock Road, Castleknock, Dublin 15, D15 YF6A, Ireland

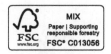

MIX
Paper | Supporting
responsible forestry
FSC
www.fsc.org   FSC® C013056

Contents

Acknowledgements

To the many parents who have contributed their ideas of how to manage their child with ADHD and gave us the insight into how to help.

To our colleagues in the local Child and Adolescent Mental Health Services teams and in the universities for their help and support. https://nfppprogram.com

This Six-Step Parenting Programme is based on the originally created New Forest Parenting Programme (NFPP) in the UK; it has been the subject of a number of research studies and has been used clinically for a number of years with a diverse range of parents; it is now used nationally and internationally to help parents.

Pages marked with ⊕ can be downloaded from https://uk.jkp.com/catalogue/book/9781805011071

PART 1

WHAT IS ADHD AND WHAT CAN WE DO ABOUT IT?

CHAPTER 1

Introduction

All children experience characteristic levels of activity. Some children are very inactive and some are hyperactive. Most professionals think about activity levels as being on a sliding scale with very inactive people at one end of the scale and very active (hyperactive) people at the other end.

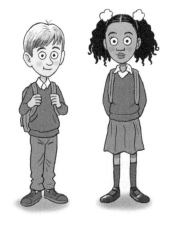

If a child's hyperactivity is causing them difficulty their parents might ask for a professional to meet with them. The child might be in trouble in playgroup or school for not concentrating or sitting down when instructed to and running around all over the place during quiet activities. The child's parents may also be finding their behaviour very difficult to manage at home. Boys and girls can present with hyperactivity in different ways.

It was thought that ADHD was more common in boys than girls, but the research tells us that in adulthood the incidence is equal. Girls present with ADHD in a different way to boys and so sometimes their difficulties can be missed. Girls often present with less hyperactivity or it appears less obvious. They can present as more inattentive, they struggle more with social interactions and organizational skills. In this book we will use the words 'they' or 'them' to indicate either gender.

When an expert in the treatment of hyperactive children, such as a nurse, health visitor or doctor, sees your child he or she may ask very specific questions about their behaviour at playgroup, school or at home. The clinician may also observe them in the clinic setting or at school; they may also conduct a computerized test of attention and concentration.

He or she may decide your child's symptoms of inattention and overactivity are severe enough for it to be possible that your child has a neurodevelopmental disorder and treatment of some kind might be suggested. The doctor or nurse might call your child's condition 'hyperactivity' or attention deficit hyperactive disorder (ADHD). For ease we will call it ADHD. ADHD is a syndrome characterized by a collection of symptoms which include hyperactivity, poor attention, and impulsivity.

ADHD is not a new disorder. It has been recognized for many years. Recent research has shown, though, how important it is to identify serious ADHD early in life. Early intervention helps children and their families to adapt their parenting approach to the particular needs of their child. Children with ADHD take much longer to learn from their parents or from the environment around them.

As parents you need to be consistent and persistent in how you help them to learn from you. Therefore it is important to start treatment as early as possible to prevent the child's behaviour becoming difficult to change, which might cause greater problems in the future. Some children who show early signs of ADHD can learn to understand their behaviour with the help of their parents and their playgroup or school and, as they get older, learn to manage these difficulties, so they become less of an issue for them.

We know that if parents can adapt their parenting to consider their child's difficulties and help the child to achieve and communicate better then their ADHD behaviours and relationships at home can improve, making time together for parent and child more fun. The child should also do better at school.

We have developed this programme of treatment which is based on what we know about children with ADHD and their families.

Understanding ADHD: What are the symptoms of ADHD?

ADHD is one of the most researched disorders of childhood. The main features of ADHD are:

- a short attention span that makes it difficult for the child to concentrate for very long

- impulsivity (which means that children cannot stop themselves from doing things)

- overactive behaviour, which shows as excessive energy that means the child is rarely still for very long.

Parents often find these features very difficult to deal with and can become very frustrated with their young child. There is often a family history of ADHD; one or other parent might have symptoms or characteristics too, which can add to the relationship difficulties.

Children with ADHD can have other difficulties as well as the three listed above. Your child may have some or all of those listed below. It might be useful to put a tick against those you see in your child, so you can remind yourself that these are part of their ADHD and not just disruptive or deliberate behaviour.

Some children with ADHD may also have poor coordination in *gross motor skills* (for example, running and playing games) and/or *fine motor skills* (such as writing or using a knife and fork). Your child with ADHD may also show some of the following signs:

- a poor short-term memory (difficulty remembering things they are asked to do)

- a very active brain, which means that they like to be kept busy

- hating to wait – therefore they will do anything to avoid waiting, even if means giving up on things they enjoy like watching a TV programme

- talking and fidgeting when they are supposed to sit quietly

- interrupting when people are talking.

Remember that each child is an individual though, and therefore the difficulties they present are unique. Children with ADHD are often very lovable children full of energy and curiosity but they can be hard work!

Children who have ADHD may also be very emotional and sensitive. People are often misled by the boisterous and active behaviour into thinking children with ADHD are emotionally tough but that is often not the case. Their ADHD behaviours and emotional sensitivity can often lead to outbursts or meltdowns that may get them into trouble. Parents and teachers can often end up in a negative battle with the child, with everyone getting upset, whereas understanding their sensitivities enables the use of more positive strategies.

The symptoms of ADHD lead to characteristic behaviours in children. Your child may for example:

- find it hard to concentrate and not be able to continue with activities such as writing or colouring for very long

- move from one activity to another without finishing anything

- rarely play for a long time, and not enjoy playing with toys or games, preferring active games

- often appear not to hear you when you speak to them – if you ask them to do something they will often forget what you have asked them to do

- have a short attention span

- fidget constantly, make noises, talk all the time

- be easily distracted by others

- be reckless, impulsive and prone to accidents.

Research has shown that children with ADHD are also at a *substantially increased risk of accidents*. It is very important that you help your child to listen when you talk about dangerous situations, for example crossing busy roads, or the importance of wearing their bicycle helmet, so that they understand the dangers, and you will need to repeat that advice on a regular basis.

The following common characteristics and problems children may have alongside their ADHD have been reported by parents and researchers:

- difficulties settling for bed and/or getting off to sleep

- waking up through the night or early in the morning

- tending to eat frequent small meals or be a faddy eater, preferring to snack if they are allowed

- a lack of social skills, being unpopular with other children and having very few, or no, friends

- frequent crying, a poor opinion of themselves, and a feeling that no one likes them

- struggling to understand, express and regulate their emotions.

ADHD exists when a child shows several of the above difficulties both at home and at school or playgroup which cause them difficulties (impairment). It is a complex disorder and children with ADHD may also have other problems, such as specific learning difficulties, aggression, anxiety or sleep problems. ADHD is also more likely to co-occur with other neurodevelopmental disorders such as autism or Tourette syndrome.

It is important to see ADHD as a developmental difficulty rather than an illness. The core features of ADHD are very common in infants, but most pre-school children gain control over attention, activity and impulsivity by the age of 4. However, it takes children with ADHD much longer. So the way your child behaves is not unusual, just unusual for their age, and they need extra help from you to learn how to control their behaviour. They may be behaving like a much younger child. It is vital that you realize that your child's problems may not improve unless you work on changing the behaviour to be more positive. This means they need to learn how to cope with the problems they have, for example difficulties with attention, activity and impulsivity. Some children may not have all three main symptoms. For example, your child may only have a very poor attention span and so it is important to assess their needs to see what you need to do to help them.

Children with ADHD are more likely to be active when they are young. As they grow older, they may grow out of their activity-related problems, but they may continue to have problems with attention and concentration, especially in school. That is why we have written this book – to help you with your child while they are young and overactive and hard work. We also suggest key ideas which will improve your child's attention and concentration and help them thrive in primary school. This programme is specifically for children up to the end of primary education.

Theories: Why children have ADHD

There are several theories regarding the causes of ADHD. We describe the main ones in this section.

ADHD is a genetic disorder and about 70% of the risk for ADHD can be explained by genes. It runs in families. It may be that there is another member of your family who is very active too, such as a parent, grandparent, brother, sister, niece or nephew. Your child may have been born with the tendency to be very overactive, impulsive or inattentive, but rest assured not all such children will go on to have major problems. Some will learn to control their behaviour with the help of their parents, playgroup leaders and teachers.

There is a lot of research into the genes that might be involved in determining whether someone might have a greater tendency to be overactive, inattentive or impulsive. Generally, the complicated research tells us that the key genes that might increase the risk of ADHD are mostly related to the neurohormone dopamine, which helps us to regulate our behaviour.

As well as genetic reasons for the condition other possible causes for ADHD are illness such as encephalitis or brain injury. In a small number of cases ADHD can also be associated with premature birth, cerebral palsy and chromosome abnormalities.

Children who have had a very difficult start in life and had adverse childhood experiences may develop symptoms of ADHD in response to this. Research has found that some children exposed to severe adverse conditions such as extreme deprivation and abusive situations might go on to have symptoms of ADHD. If your child has experienced this, the strategies will still help but you might need extra support from professionals to treat the trauma alongside their ADHD, so seek help if you feel you need to.

The brain in children with ADHD

Research suggests that parts of the brain in children with ADHD work less efficiently than the brains of children without the disorder. The brain works like an electrical circuit, with neurones connecting the brain and parts of the body. For example, when a person decides they want to raise their hand, a signal is sent from the frontal cortex in the brain to the motor cortex, this signal then runs along the neurone to the specific part of the brain that controls the relevant muscles. A signal is sent back down the hand and the hand will be raised. The different neurones involved connect through junctions called synapses, and chemicals are needed to bridge the 'synaptic gap' between the neurones to pass the message on.

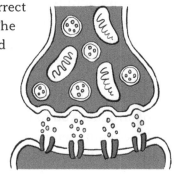

Children with ADHD seem to lack the correct balance of chemicals in these gaps. The chemical that seems to be lacking is called dopamine. This means that signals are not carried correctly, and the signals may be carried to the wrong part of the brain (like a train sent off on the wrong track at a junction). This may mean that the child will become impulsive and not be able to stop shouting, for example, as the signal to stop shouting is not working.

Because the brain may not be working as well as it should and may not send messages to the correct part of the brain, other problems may appear as well, such as problems with listening. Often, children with ADHD find it difficult to hold eye contact, which means it is hard to get their attention. They also find it hard to maintain attention and therefore easily become distracted. They may flit from game to game, and from task to task. It is hard to get them to sit still and finish a game with you. We call this 'going off task'.

If you ask a child with ADHD to do something, they may forget what you have asked them to do because they have a poor short-term memory. Being organized is also hard, because children with ADHD have problems with planning and carrying out tasks that need to be done in a sequence, like getting up in the morning, putting on clothes, brushing teeth and so on. Thus not only will they get distracted from tasks, but they will find that remembering to do them all in the right order is also difficult.

As we have said, your child may find it hard to control their impulsive behaviour. So they may get cross easily and hit out. Or they will run off and may be more likely to have accidents. Some children may have problems waiting and may appear as if they are bored easily. They might find it hard to get motivated to start tasks, to pay attention and to do what you have asked them to do.

Neuropsychological difficulties in ADHD

So why do children with ADHD behave in the way that they do (inattention, overactivity, impulsivity and distractibility). Why does ADHD not make your child tidy, motivated to learn and anxious to help you around the house? The answer lies in part in the neuroscience of ADHD, which could fill this entire book, but we are going to introduce you to the basics in just a page. Essentially there are three neuroscientific reasons that explain why children with ADHD behave in the way that they do.

1. *Executive functioning* This involves higher order cognitive processes that the ADHD child is essentially less good at because the brains of children with ADHD tend work less efficiently. Executive functioning includes *planning*: do you have to plan for your ADHD child, do they lose book bags, school jumpers and water bottles? It also includes *working memory,* the part of your memory system that helps you to remember things for long enough until your brain decides whether it needs to remember the memory. We can't remember everything – some things, like bad smells, we don't want to remember. Working memory allows us to remember things strategically. However children with ADHD have a lower capacity in their

working memory and when it becomes overloaded memories are forgotten before the brain can work out whether they are important or not. The last key component of executive functioning is *inhibitory control*. This is what stops us from responding when we should not respond. Two children, one with ADHD and one without, might climb up on to a high wall to jump off for fun. The inhibitory control system of the child without ADHD would warn them not to jump as it was too high. For the child with ADHD, their inhibitory control system would work less efficiently and would warn them not to jump just as they were falling to the ground, they would land hard on their ankle and have another trip to A&E!

2. *Motivation to wait* (also called delay aversion) Children with ADHD find waiting deeply unpleasant and almost painful. So when they experience waiting they are often motivated to avoid having to wait. How the child responds to waiting depends on how much control they have over their environment. When playing with friends where they have a lot of control they will often choose to give up on play (which looks impulsive). In situations where they have very little control, such as in the classroom, they quickly learn that they can't leave the classroom, so instead will distract themselves from the waiting by daydreaming, fidgeting or being disruptive. See below for an example you can share with family and friends.

3. *Time* is the last neuroscience example. To put it simply children with ADHD don't understand time; they can't estimate time and can't reproduce intervals of time because time means very little to them. This is important because we live in a world which is run by time, and everyone else talks in intervals of time: 'wait a minute' or 'I will be with you in five minutes'. Children with ADHD often interrupt, intrude and pester their parents and other adults not because they want to make them cross but because they either can't wait any longer or because they think they have waited for five minutes as they have been asked to do, even if it has only been thirty seconds.

This diagram shows how motivation to avoid delay might influence how your child behaves in different settings.

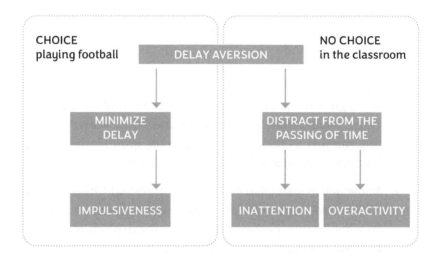

Associated problems with ADHD

As well as the main characteristics of ADHD there are usually *associated problems*, which may be the cause of much parental anger and frustration.

Examples of the associated behaviours exhibited by your child with ADHD may include:

- insatiability, including constant whingeing
- food fads – they tend to 'graze' rather than enjoy proper meals
- difficulty in getting to bed and getting to sleep
- noisiness – they may talk constantly from morning to night
- a lack of understanding of social skills – they tend to invade other people's space and find it difficult to be aware of other people's needs
- difficulty in taking turns and sharing

- difficulty making and keeping friends, for example they may be less likely to be invited to other children's parties

- they may have significant mood swings, with good days and bad days and, possibly, good weeks and bad weeks

- emotional immaturity – they may be at only about two-thirds of the emotional age of their peers

- dislike of change – such as a change of daily routine or a change of carer or teacher

- learning difficulties are frequently present – it is thought that between 40 and 60 per cent of children with ADHD have learning problems, such as difficulty with reading, writing and numerical skills

- problems with language may occur, with understanding others and sometimes with expressing themselves – sometimes these problems can be very subtle and take some effort to remedy.

Children with ADHD who are also temperamentally sensitive

Some children with ADHD are also what is known as 'temperamentally sensitive'. In referring to temperament we mean a child's nature, make-up, the way they respond in different situations. Children's temperaments range from easy at one end to difficult at the other. Easy children are quick to calm down when upset, are not very fussy and tend to 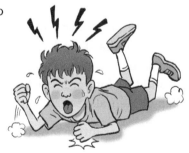 be happy-go-lucky. Children who are temperamentally sensitive, on the other hand, are not easy to calm down, they may be very fussy, they always want things done a certain way and they may get upset at the slightest thing.

The characteristics of temperamentally difficult children include:

- They may have been a difficult baby who was hard to soothe.

- They may not have a regular body rhythm, sleeping poorly.

- They get upset easily and react very strongly when upset.

- They get upset about minor things.

- They dislike change and take time to get used to new situations.

- They can be a fussy, difficult feeder.

- They can be very demanding.

- They may have low self-esteem.

These children tend to get their own way a lot. It may be that parents will give in to them for a quiet life, as whining and crying are exhausting to live with. This could make your relationship with your child unhappy and it you may not feel properly in charge. It is likely that your child will not feel very happy either. Children can feel very unsafe about having a lot of control.

As a parent you may feel that nothing you do will be enough, as your child moans at the end of treats and always wants to stay longer or to have another go. Temperamentally sensitive children are very hard work for parents, who inevitably get impatient and may become very critical. Below we provide a list of general hints and tips for parents whose children have ADHD and are also temperamentally sensitive.

- It is important for you as a parent to accept the child that you have. The child's temperament is the way it is and if you adjust your parenting style to suit it life can become much more enjoyable for the whole family.

- Routines and structure are particularly important for sensitive children.

- Children who have sensitive temperaments need some space and peace in their day.

- Clear boundaries are fundamental. Work out which rules are important and which are not. Once you have decided which ones are important, be consistent in expecting those rules to be followed. For example, safety rules are important but it may not be worth having battles over what your child wears!

- Avoid angry confrontations as much as possible. With ADHD children defusing a situation early is the best option.

- Improve your child's listening skills. Keep your instructions short and clear. Maintain eye contact by gently holding the child's head if necessary.

- Improve your child's self-esteem by using praise as much as possible when it is appropriate. Warm touches can be helpful here; a stroke or a pat as your child goes past you can be very important. Cuddles and loving touches, even massage, are also helpful to soothe this kind of child. End the day on a positive note.

Understanding that many children with behaviour difficulties associated with ADHD have a very short fuse can help us to avoid some potential pitfalls. It is important to know that the child's outbursts are not deliberate but part of their inner emotional make-up, which they did not choose.

Professionals working with children with behaviour problems have noticed that sometimes when a child has a fragile temperament this can lead to difficulties with behavioural and social interactions in adulthood. It has also been shown that a difficult temperament at age 7, combined with a lack of consistent family behaviour rules, is strongly associated with significant behaviour problems in the teen years (even worse than normal).

The child with ADHD, as we know, often has the triple burdens of impulsivity, hyperactivity and inattention. In addition to this the child may well be temperamentally fragile. This has important implications for all those who deal with or live with such children. The way that a parent, teacher or carer handles testing behaviours will depend on how well he or she understands the child's emotional make-up.

Children with ADHD have strengths too

In the process of understanding about children with ADHD you might feel that everything is really difficult and struggle to see any positives. However there are many positives to having a child with ADHD, and children with ADHD often have the following strengths of character and show the following positive behaviours:

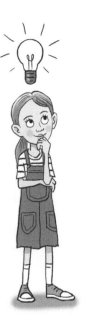

- They have lots of energy to play and have fun with.

- They may be creative and can work out new things quickly.

- They may have quick reflexes and do well at sport.

- They can think around problems and ways to adapt to new situations when appropriate.

- They can develop alternative ways of learning.

- They can act quickly when you need them to.

- They think differently and can be a step ahead of those around them.

- When they focus, they achieve a lot.

- They can have an amazing imagination.

- They are tenacious (they keep going even when others would have given up).

- They can have a great sense of humour.

- They can be kind and caring towards others.

Just as we have noticed the difficulties a child with ADHD might have, it is equally important to notice all the good things they do and keep acknowledging these. The 'stories' children hear about themselves are important to their self-esteem and their future, so make sure you are pointing out all their strengths!

Despite the strengths of a child with ADHD some of the characteristics associated with it can be a real problem that affects children and families. Parents do their best and what you are doing is probably already pretty good, but it may need some fine tuning to make it work for your child with ADHD. What seem to be little changes can make an enormous difference. Increasing your knowledge about ADHD and following the steps outlined in this book will help you to understand and anticipate what is happening. In this book we present tried and tested strategies to help parents. We know from other colleagues' work and research studies that the strategies suggested in this book will work. The techniques themselves are not particularly difficult, but you may well find remembering to do them hard at first. We suggest that you have someone, a partner, friend or parent, who may help you and offer some support over the next few weeks while you work through the programme.

CHAPTER 2

Parenting a Child with ADHD

The importance of adapting (tailoring) your parenting

As we have said before, parenting children with ADHD can be hard work. In this book we will work with you to try to rethink your parenting toward your child and think of your child in a different way. We hope that you will understand that your child is not deliberately trying to misbehave, or get back at you, and that it is important that you don't take your child's behaviour personally.

As you know it is important that you try to accept the child you have. The child's ADHD and temperament are part of your child's make-up that they were born with. When you adjust your parenting style to your child, life becomes more pleasant for you and your family.

Parents will be the key in bringing about changes for the better in their child's behaviour and social development. It is the parent who will have to adopt the appropriate strategies to effect improvement in their child's behaviour as the child is too young to do this for themselves – they need you to help them.

What affects your parenting?

Parenting a child with significant behaviour problems is emotionally and physically draining. Parents' feelings of being deskilled by the child and feeling they are being blamed for their child's behaviour may create ripple effects impacting on the parents, the marriage, other siblings, the extended family and the community.

One parent may feel angry if their partner denies the problem or withdraws from the situation. One parent may have an easier relationship with the child and this, too, can lead to resentment. If the mum is the main carer, the husband/partner can feel that he is being excluded by the constant attention given to the misbehaving child, and the same applies to brothers and sisters.

Parents of children with behaviour problems are often (perhaps usually) blamed by lay people and professionals alike. They are given the message that their child's problem could have been solved if only the parent had been 'more this, or more that'. Other parents who have had children without behaviour problems feel certain that the affected parent is inadequate. These lucky parents may be very insensitive to those who have problems. This reinforces the sense of helplessness experienced by parents of a child with any difficulties.

How we have been parented ourselves influences our parenting and it is important to seek help if you don't feel you are parenting as you want to.

You may not feel it, but people working with families and children with hyperactivity do understand the difficulties you may be experiencing. We acknowledge that, and know it is very hard work. It is not your fault or your child's fault. You are probably doing well under difficult circumstances and other parents may have it easier.

Parents with ADHD themselves

Parents of children with ADHD may have ADHD themselves. This means they may find sticking to the strategies difficult as they struggle with planning, organization, consistency and memory. If you have ADHD symptoms, finding a mentor to support you as you go through the programme can help; we talk more about this later in the book.

What you can do to help your child

We know a lot, through research and experience sharing, about the kind of parenting which works best for all children, and especially the style of parenting and strategies which work best for children with ADHD. The best results for ADHD children are when a parent can adjust their parenting to the needs of their child, which may not be easy.

Parents need to communicate and negotiate clearly with their child with ADHD so the child can understand what the parent wants them to do. The child should be able to understand the rules of the house. Rules should be consistent and fair with lots of praise for good behaviour and appropriate consequences for behaviour that is not acceptable. The rules, praise and consequences should be appropriate to the age of the child and be respectful to the child and workable. Parenting can be fun a lot of the time but doing it right is hard work and requires commitment and the investment of time.

The long-term goal is for your child to learn to control their behaviour with the support of you, as their parents, and their teachers and to grow up feeling good about themselves, with the adults they interact with appreciating their positive points.

We hope that by explaining to you why children with ADHD find aspects of life hard it will be easier for you to understand why they behave the way they do. This will help you to understand why children who are like this need to be parented differently. We hope that this will make it easier for you to be more positive in your approach to parenting your child with ADHD and to understand why they behave this way. This should also make you feel more in control. For example, when a child with ADHD doesn't listen it is not because they are ignoring you but because they find it difficult and effortful to listen. We will suggest ways to gain your child's attention in order to begin to try to change their behaviour. Children with ADHD have real difficulty in organizing their lives so we will suggest strategies that can help.

Behaviour strategies are helpful for children with ADHD. These are ideas to help parents manage their child's difficult behaviour. As we have said, we know that effective and informed parenting of children with ADHD is very important in preventing the child from becoming oppositional and aggressive. We also know that *parenting is extremely hard work,* and this is why presenting simple behaviour strategies for parents to follow is usually the first approach.

It may feel to you as parents that you are going over things you may have tried in the past with little success. Understanding the characteristics of ADHD will help you to distinguish those behaviours that the child cannot help from those which you as parents can help to change.

Changing your parenting approach can be difficult. We have used the ideas we present in this book in our clinic, in groups and individual sessions, and the tried and tested advice in the book has helped many families in several countries. *With a new approach parents often see a big difference in their child's behaviour.*

Below we list some pointers to remember. They will help you to help your child.

- Your child will find it difficult to control their symptoms of ADHD and will find it hard to concentrate and pay attention.

- Nobody is to blame for your child's condition.

- ADHD often runs in families, so you may notice some of the characteristics in family members, or even yourself!

- Adapting your parenting and using the strategies we describe brings about real change in most cases.

- Children with ADHD take longer to learn things from you so you need to be consistent and persistent to help them.

It is important to realize that change very rarely occurs overnight. It will usually take a few months to see a significant improvement. It will probably be hard work but worth it in the long run – changing your parenting approach can be difficult. As far as possible make sure that all the adults who look after your child agree to adopt the same approach to handling their behaviour, and do so in broadly the same way, as *consistency is very important.*

Many families of children with ADHD understandably feel guilty, anxious and angry. Parents may well feel worn out and depressed. Their child may be shunned by friends and neighbours and their behaviour in public can be so embarrassing that the parent avoids social contact outside the home.

There are, of course, different degrees of ADHD and the behaviour of each affected child will be slightly different. The presence of ADHD in a particular child only becomes a problem when their behaviour is unacceptable to others and/or problematic to them. Parents may have managed the pre-school child without noticing a problem until they attend playschool or school, for example. The alarmed parent may then be informed that the playschool or school cannot cope with their child.

ADHD in its extreme form can appear at different stages. Gross motor hyperactivity (like running around) can change to fidgeting and restlessness for example, as the child must conform to sitting down for long periods in the school setting. Fidgeting is thus more noticeable in older children.

Understanding behaviour, the New Forest Parenting Programme (NFPP) processes helping parents to help their child

In this step-by-step book we recognize that when children with ADHD are experiencing difficulties there are often a number of explanations that can be used to make sense of their behaviour alongside their ADHD difficulties. We use these to help you to understand your own child's behaviour; this then forms the basis of the 'tool kit' of ideas to help you to help your child.

- Biological theories: we explain why your child might be over-active, the roles of genetics and how the interaction between genes and environment can be used to help your child. We explore with you your child's temperament and suggest ideas to improve their attention by using attention training and 'delay restructuring' ideas – all these really help the 'active child'.

- Psychodynamic theories: we consider how you and your child's relationship has formed over the years and how this has been influenced by your own experiences of being parented, as well as your child's temperament. We explore with you how to be able to see things from your child's view-point and to really observe and understand why behaviours might happen – even if they are not aware of why.

- Cognitive theories: how you or your child's thoughts, feelings and beliefs may be influencing your behaviours and whether these beliefs are helpful to you both.

- Behavioural theories: behaviour management, rewards, reinforcement, looking at what might be reinforcing a behaviour and giving ideas to help.

- Systemic approaches: thinking together about your unique family system, how you work together, how you can be curious about what is happening and what function a behaviour might be serving in the family. We help you to look out for unhelpful repeating patterns; using others' thoughts about what is happening we work with you to think about having consistency across settings so that your child is clear on what is expected.

The New Forest Parenting Programme principles

This book has been written as a result of many years of research and working with families trying out and testing ideas that parents have found useful. In addition to this our knowledge of ADHD has expanded and we understand better the underlying difficulties within the brain the child with ADHD may experience. It is with this in mind that we have developed the principles behind the programme, which we translate into action step-by-step.

The techniques themselves are not particularly difficult, but you may well find them to be hard work at first. We suggest that you have someone, a partner, friend or parent, who may help you and offer some support over the next six steps. Many parents do their best and what you are doing is probably pretty good, but it may need some 'fine tuning' to make it work for your child with ADHD. Knowledge about ADHD will help you to see what is happening.

Principle 1: To help parents to really understand ADHD and how it affects their child

First, it is important to help you as a parent accept the child that you have and that you really understand what ADHD is. Children with ADHD are unique and this means that their difficulties can be unique to them. Parents need to observe their child so that they can see which particular difficulties they are experiencing. This may seem obvious, but it involves you really observing your child and really acknowledging what they genuinely have difficulty with, and how they cope in certain situations.

Alongside this, parents need to consider their child's temperament – are they quiet and shy or outgoing and boisterous, do they whinge and cry or are they passive and accepting? How does their temperament compare to others within the family? For example, if a mother is very anxious generally is the child the same? In which case, by acknowledging your similarities (or differences) it might help you to adjust your parenting style to calm the child and life can become much nicer for the whole family.

Once you can acknowledge their ADHD symptoms and the type of temperament they have and what adaptions you may have to make, then moving on to the next principle of the programme becomes easier. Your relationship with your child is crucial to their well-being and it might well have been under strain without you really understanding why. By understanding their ADHD behaviours, which are not their fault or yours, we hope that you can rebuild your relationship knowing what behaviours your child can change and what behaviours result from their ADHD and they need your help with.

Principle 2: To provide you with a 'tool kit' of ideas that you can use every day with your child

This involves behaviour strategies; these have been developed taking into account the neuropsychological difficulties seen in some children with ADHD, for example short-term memory problems, difficulty with waiting, poor organizational skills and so on.

We will give you suggestions to help you as parents manage your children's difficult behaviours relating to their ADHD. As we have said, we know that effective and informed parenting of children with ADHD is very important in preventing them from becoming oppositional and aggressive. We also know that parenting is *extremely hard work*, and this is why behaviour strategies are one of the first approaches.

We advise you to use the diaries in this book to help you understand why certain situations occur. The diaries are for both positive and difficult times. Using diaries can sometimes help you to see patterns emerging, for example if a certain behaviour happens at the same time each day or at a certain place you can look in depth at the lead up to the situation and use strategies to help alter it.

With the positive diary you can see what is working and how to do more!

Principle 3: To focus on helping your child improve their attention through play

Assess your child's abilities, initially through play, in preparation for attention training to improve concentration, working memory, waiting and so on.

We will ask you to observe what your child is like when they are asked to do something. We will encourage you to work out exactly what your child can do in order to have a positive starting place. We call this *scoping* the child's abilities.

We will encourage you to increase the difficulty of the tasks as the child masters each stage. We call this *extending* the child's abilities. For example, we might ask you to observe how long your child can concentrate for. We will then ask you to play with your child for that length of time and encourage them to concentrate all that time. When you think they can do that we will ask you to encourage them to concentrate for one minute longer and so on.

We will ask you to encourage the child in such a way that they feel positive about the help they are getting. We would like you to think about how you can help them so they feel in charge and can work out what to do with your help. You will try to help them in such a way that you are not stepping in and doing it for them or taking over. You are *holding* them through change. We call this *scaffolding* (just like the scaffolding that holds up a building allowing the different floors to be put on).

We will encourage you to do this in the home and then to take the skills outside the home. We call this *generalizing*. We will encourage the use of *teachable moments* to use these new skills in school, at granny's, in the supermarket and so on. We apply this initially through the medium of play but expand this to other situations through the programme.

Playing with your child has added benefits in that it can help you reform your relationship if things have been tough between you. It helps to improve self-esteem, to learn new skills, learn to share and take turns, and can really help to expand language and communication skills.

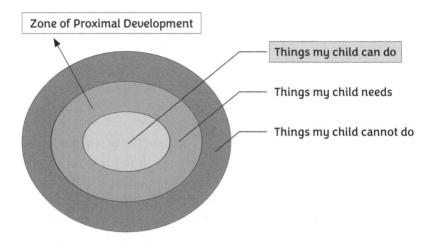

Principle 4: To help your child learn to understand feelings and control their emotions

Understanding that many children with behaviour difficulties associated with ADHD have a very 'short fuse' can help us to avoid some potential pitfalls. It is important to know that these outbursts are not deliberate but part of the child's innate emotional make-up, which they did not choose!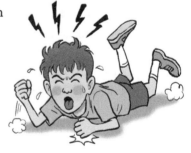

Professionals working with children with behaviour problems have noticed that childhood temperamental fragility can lead to difficulties with behavioural and social interactions later in adulthood. It has also been shown that a difficult temperament at age 7, combined with a lack of consistent family behaviour rules, is strongly associated with significant behaviour problems in the teen years.

The child with ADHD, as we know, has the triple burdens of impulsivity, hyperactivity and inattention. As we have already suggested, in *addition* to this, the child may well be temperamentally fragile. This has important implications for all those who deal with or live with such a child. Thus the way that a parent, teacher or carer handles testing behaviours will depend on how well they understand the child's emotional make-up.

Principle 5: To transfer what you have learned to others and use ideas when outside the home

Having practised all the principles yourself, usually at home, the important skill is to share these with other people involved in the care of your child and to practise them outside the home. So having strategies that work in supermarkets or when you are on an outing is important for the social life of your family. We recommend trying the principles at home first then, once you have mastered them and your child is beginning to understand the rules, try them outside the home. The programme provides you with a 'tool kit' of ideas to call upon when difficult situations arise; examples include using mindfulness, Social Stories or considering sensory difficulties.

Principle five also includes making sure that everyone (the whole system) involved in caring for your child understands what is needed to help them succeed, despite their ADHD difficulties, and becomes their advocate – educating others about your child and their needs is key to this. We are all in a relationship with each other and how we react will influence how others react to us, and vice versa, so it is important to consider how understanding and supportive the 'system' (family, school, friends and so on) is to help your child with ADHD.

Principle 6: What to do when times are tough

What do you do when times are tough? Due to the genetic aspect of ADHD it is likely there are others within the family having similar difficulties and, even if you can't immediately identify with this, all families have times when life is more difficult.

Throughout the programme we focus on helping parents to value how important their physical and mental health is to their child's well-being and how important their parenting is for their child.

> What is happening in your life will contribute to how much energy you have to parent so your well-being is crucial.

A recent bereavement, divorce, marital problem, financial problem or mental or physical health problem may make it extremely difficult for a parent to put these ideas into practice. Your own experience of being parented may also impact on how you parent your child, sometimes without you realizing the impact it is having.

Personalizing the programme to meet your family's needs

You may need to adapt the programme to suit you and your partner's background. As discussed below, in some cultures a child making eye contact with an adult in a position of authority is not thought to be respectful, so if this is the case you will need to find other ways of making sure your child is listening to you, especially when you want to praise them. Your religion or culture may not allow the playing of cards (one of the games we suggest for practising working on attention and concentration). If this is so, find other games that do the same task and play them instead.

You may be someone who finds concentration difficult yourself; be fair to yourself and give yourself small 'win-win' (achievable) goals to work on. For example, 'Today I will work on getting them to give me eye contact to make sure they are listening, and I will praise them when they do this. Tomorrow I will carry on doing that and work on...'.

Summary

Children with ADHD need a different kind of parenting.

- It is important to start changes in parenting as early as possible to teach the child new skills and to prevent the child's behaviour from causing them ongoing problems.

- It is fundamental that you recognize that this is not your child's fault. They are the way they are as they were born this way. This will help you begin to accept the child you have.

- Some children who present with early signs of ADHD can be helped to learn to contain their symptoms with the help of parents and the playgroup or school so that the symptoms may be less of a problem for them as they get older.

- We know that if parents can adapt their parenting to their child and help the child to learn to control their behaviour relationships at home will be better and more fun for parents and children.

- The parent may be parenting well but the parenting will need 'fine tuning' to adapt to the ADHD child. This will aid the child's entry to school.

- We believe that if we can help you parent your child differently than you can help them learn to cope better with their problems with ADHD. We will teach you to be your child's trainer.

- You will find it easier to deal with them and they will get into trouble less. This will help you feel even more skilled in helping them and make your time together more fun and rewarding.

CHAPTER 3

Getting Ready for the Step-by-Step Programme

Further considerations

Remember that there will be good days and some not so good days. This is normal. Sometimes events will go well and sometimes they will not. Just start again the next day if events have not gone well – do not give up. In each step of the programme we will ask you to review how the previous step has gone, considering what has been successful and what has not. This will help you consider how to change your approach, if necessary.

When you fine tune how you manage and carry out instructions, do expect that your child may well appear worse for the first few days. This is because they are used to old ways and change is difficult for them too. The aim is for you, the parents, to understand what is happening, and for us to give you ideas that can help you cope and to improve your child's behaviour.

We know that the ideas we give you might be easy to read but less easy to put into practice. Yet it does work (eventually!). Most people do not have lessons on child-rearing – they must learn as they go along and often repeat the pattern of their own parents' child-rearing techniques, for better or for worse.

Parents are often worried that 'treating' ADHD will make the child lose their 'spark'. It may be the so-called spark, however, that is causing heartache for one parent. The other parent may feel that there is no problem and say, 'they are fine with me'. This can sometimes be explained by the fact that seeing one parent if they work full time is a comparative rarity and the child may behave better with them. Whoever is the main caregiver is more 'familiar' to the child. In contrast, a different parent may spend only a small part of the day with the child, and the child will view playing and reading and other activities with them as a novelty. The same principle may be seen with grandparents and uncles and aunts, and other adults, so the child behaves better with them than they do with their main caregiver. This may make parents feel insecure about their parenting skills, especially when other adults find it difficult to believe that there is a problem with the child's behaviour.

It is important for the family to understand that the earlier help is given the easier it is to achieve good results. One parent might recognize the difficulties but they might be less obvious to the other parent. School may recognize the difficulties and make it easier for the parents to reach an agreement.

Some parents would prefer a 'wait and see' approach. The fact is that the sooner help is offered the easier it is to improve behaviour. With every year that goes by without appropriate intervention it becomes more difficult to bring about change.

> The most important factor of all, which appears in all six steps, is: if your child feels valued, worthwhile, approved of and you can spend time with them, they will feel loved and respected.

Learning styles

It is important to understand your child's learning style (as well as your own). Each of us finds some ways of learning easier than others, for example some people learn best when they are shown things, some when they are told things, some when they read things and some when they do it themselves.

If you try one approach and it doesn't seem to be working, try a different learning style – it may not be the approach not working, just the way you are trying to get your child to learn it from you! Sometimes a combination of learning styles is needed. Remember too, play is one of the best ways to learn!

Diet

The evidence on the effect of diet on children's behaviour has been increasing recently and many parents have told us that certain sweets seem to affect their child's behaviour. Two studies have shown that this is possible. The first looked at artificial colours and preservatives, a certain number of these increased children's activity levels. This is especially important if your child is already active as it might increase the level of activity further.[1] Another study looked at the role of Omega 3 and 6 oils in helping children's attention and suggested supplementing with these was effective to some degree.[2] There is also some evidence that if your child has a learning or reading difficulty they might be helped by supplementation.[3]

Diet in itself is important, for example a breakfast that has no fat, no protein and a high glycaemic index (high level of processed sugar) causes the blood sugar to rise. This then causes the body to increase the amount of circulating insulin to break down the high level of sugars. The blood sugar then crashes as the insulin breaks down the sugar, this triggers the release of a stress hormone: adrenaline.

Adrenaline makes the child fidgety and inattentive. If your child already has the difficulties associated with ADHD this could make them worse.

It is therefore important that your child has a well-balanced diet, which is high in nutrients and contains plenty of fresh fruit and vegetables as well as oily fish. As far as possible sugar should be obtained from complex carbohydrates, which have a much slower absorption avoiding the influx of insulin, such as bananas or porridge.

Many of the low calorie, low in sugar drinks seen on supermarket shelves contain additives – it is worth avoiding these and replacing with water, milk or diluted fresh juice. Making fruit smoothies together can be a good way of getting children to have a range of fruit. Homemade vegetable soups are cheap and easy to make and a way of disguising vegetables that children may not like. It is important to remember that sometimes children need to try something 10 times before they like it, while their taste buds get used to it. It is also important to occasionally retry things we may not have liked, as our tastes change as we get older.

> It is important that you take care of your nutrition too; you are very important to your child's welfare and if you are unwell then your ability to care for them is reduced. So eat well – together!

Sleep problems

We know a lot of children with ADHD also have problems with settling to sleep and staying asleep. Some children also get up very early too. Research has informed us that this is probably to do with melatonin production in the brain. Melatonin is a chemical produced by the brain as night falls and is responsible for telling the brain that it is time to go to sleep. In children with ADHD the production of this hormone is delayed. In addition, modern appliances using 'bright light' such as computer or gaming systems may delay melatonin production further.

Sleep is very important for all children; it helps them process information learned during the day. If a child doesn't get enough sleep, this processing is less effective. This means you might be working hard at getting them to understand something but it is never consolidated by the brain.

Good sleep routines are essential to help the child with ADHD. Before tackling your child's sleep issues it is important remember to prepare a child for an event, for example warning a child (e.g. before bed time) with lots of prompts and/or planned routines that remind a child that this is the routine that will finish up with going to bed, e.g. tea time, play time, bath time, story, cuddle, sleep; gradually making bed time earlier and cueing, e.g. establishing a bedtime routine with good effect, for example gradually reducing the amount of attention given by parents to a child waking during the night; reinforcement for desired behaviour such as staying in bed, using star charts for praise.

Example 1: Johnny will not go to bed

The parents have got so tired that they let him go to sleep down-stairs, then they carry him upstairs. Check that you, the parents, are feeling strong and ready for working on the sleep issues.

Discuss setting a bed routine and bedtime. (You may have to work toward this.) For example:

- Tea at the same time, e.g. 5 pm.

- After tea play with a parent for half an hour, 5.30 to 6 pm (not computer games or TV).

- Bath/wash time at 6 pm.

- Into bed: read a story (decide in advance how long you will read for).

- Cover toys and say good night to him.

- Then give him a kiss and stay with him. Do not speak to him, (read a book or a magazine).

- If he always gets up, sit and hold his hand till he falls asleep. He has to stay in his own bed – reward with a star for staying in bed

- Do that for *three* nights.

- Then tell him that you will sit with him but not touch him.

- Do that for the next *three* nights.

- Then gradually tell him that you will stay in the room but not sit beside him.

- Then gradually move out to be in the hall, and if the child calls out ignore him.

- The child will then get rewards for staying in his own bed.

Parents need to be strong and will need support.

Example 2: Mary comes into her parents' bed at night

Parents have tried to put her back into her bed, but she will not stay.

- When parents are feeling strong, take her back to her own bed.

- Tell her what is happening. Set rules for getting up, e.g. smiley face on parents' bedroom door when she can come in, neutral face when she has to stay out.

- Agree rewards with her for staying in her own bed.

Setting boundaries and rules around electronic games, phones and so on is really important – a rule of no games or phones in the bedroom can help in teenage years if started when your child is young!

The Six-Step Parenting Programme

Children with ADHD need a different approach to parenting than children without ADHD. This programme aims to give you a 'tool kit' of ideas you can try with your child. If you try these ideas out and practise them, you will find that you and your child will get along better.

We have developed a simple treatment programme that you can work through yourself at your own pace. When we use the programme in clinics with families they work through it a week at a time, but some families progress more quickly and others take more time. What is important is to realize that it will not produce instant change but will over time give you more confidence and provide you with ideas which work for children with ADHD. Practice, more practice and consistency will produce real detectable changes in your child's behaviour and attitude.

As we have already said, the Six-Step Parenting Programme is based on the New Forest Parenting Programme, an evidence-based intervention for parents of children with ADHD that has been evaluated and implemented around the world. In some cultures particular strategies may be difficult to administer. For example, some parents may find using eye contact for positive interactions difficult as their cultural beliefs may mean that a child making eye contact with an adult is not permitted. If you come across a strategy that you find difficult, rather than not use it, try to find a way to adapt it to meet the aim of the six steps within your cultural or personal beliefs. For example, instead of eye contact, touch could be used to signify that the child should listen, and then praise could be given. This would reinforce that the child needs to listen carefully and receive positive feedback, which in turn enables them to listen more and increases their self-esteem. As you will see in Step 1 this is the aim of eye contact in this strategy. For further details of the evaluation of NFPP including evaluation of this self-help version please visit our website https://nfppprogram.com.

The programme is organized into six steps. We suggest that you work through the material over the next few weeks, reading and concentrating on *one step at a time.* Try out the ideas we have suggested in that step for managing your own child's ADHD symptoms. When you are comfortable with the ideas and confident they are working in practice *move on to the next step.* As you move on, keep practising the previous steps, if necessary going back to the elements that are not working so well for you and your child.

At each step the programme will give you something new to work on and suggest you practise it as much as you can. We will also suggest games to play with your child that will help them improve their attention. Most of these games involve using a traditional pack of cards, which is cheap to buy and easy to carry around. We will give you ideas to help your child learn to wait for longer and not be so impatient. We will make practical suggestions that will help your child learn to organize themselves better.

The most important aspect of the programme is when we explain to you why a child with ADHD behaves the way they do, so that you can understand that your child's behaviour is the way it is because they have underlying problems, not because they are naughty.

They might, for example, have problems listening, paying attention or waiting their turn.

There will be, of course, times when your child, like any other child, might just be being naughty, so we will help you learn to identify when that might be the case so you can deal with that too. The fundamental point, though, is that children who have ADHD have real problems that underlie much of their behaviour and are not, in the main, deliberately being naughty.

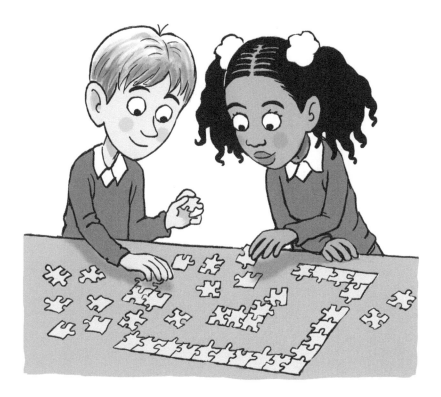

Notes

1   McCann, D., Barrett, A., Cooper, A., Crumpler, D., *et al.* (2007) Food additives and hyperactive behaviour in 3-year-old and 8/9-year-old children in the community: a randomised, double-blinded, placebo-controlled trial. *The Lancet*, 370(9598), 1560–7.

2   Johnson, M., Östlund, S., Fransson, G., Kadesjö, B., & Gillberg, C. (2009) Omega-3/ omega-6 fatty acids for attention deficit hyperactivity disorder: a randomized placebo-controlled trial in children and adolescents. *Journal of Attention Disorders*, 12(5), 394–401.

3   Johnson, M., Fransson, G., Östlund, S., Areskoug, B., & Gillberg, C. (2017) Omega 3/6 fatty acids for reading in children: a randomized, double-blind, placebo-controlled trial in 9-year-old mainstream schoolchildren in Sweden. *Journal of Child Psychology and Psychiatry*, 58(1), 83–93.

PART 2

THE SIX-STEP PROGRAMME FOR HELPING YOUR CHILD WITH ADHD

Introduction

Where do we start?

Before you embark on the stages in the six-step programme we suggest that you make sure you are familiar with the ideas about ADHD we have outlined in the first part of the book. If you are unsure of ADHD symptoms then have another look at the opening chapter. It is important that you understand those behaviours that your child cannot help and those they need help with.

Then you should read the ideas from the first step. Once you think you are ready, then move on to step two and onwards. In each step there are tasks that we wish you to study and to put into practice.

The steps need to be carried out in the order in the book, as the early ones provide the foundations for those that follow. The first step helps you understand and adjust to your child's ADHD behaviours. The next step outlines strategies to help children with ADHD. The third step shows you how to improve your child's attention through play activities. Communication is fundamental, and the fourth step outlines ways you can improve the ways you and your child communicate. The fifth step gives practical guidance on managing your ADHD child outside the home. The sixth and final step indicates ways forward when your child faces school or other important life transitions, and recaps what you have learned through the programme.

Within the book you can review the skills and tasks by using diaries and we suggest that you reflect on tasks by talking to your partner or friend as you go along. Some of the things we suggest may seem very repetitive but bear with us, as these will help you build on your skills over time and practice will help you to be more confident.

Parents with symptoms of ADHD themselves

We are asking you to be organized, to anticipate and to plan ahead so you can become your child's trainer. This may be difficult for you to do, however it is not impossible. This is a simple six-step programme we have used with many families. You can take as short or as long a time as you need to work through the stages in this book.

What we have found is that parents who have symptoms of ADHD themselves often need a little longer to first master the tasks for themselves before they can then help their child. This is fine. Do not lose heart; it is harder for you to do these things, but you will get there in the end.

Work steadily at mastering a task then move on.

Seek someone who can review with you how you are doing. Sometimes if you have ADHD yourself you might find it hard to be patient. For example, you have asked your child to do something and he does not do it immediately. Try not to be impulsive and allow yourself to get cross. Try to wait until he has a chance to do it. We think that a parent should try to wait at least *five seconds* to allow the child with ADHD to respond to your request (the *five second rule*) before jumping in and becoming cross.

If your child does not do what you have asked them to do, gently remind them what it is that you want them to do. Remember to make sure you have eye contact when appropriate, and check your child is listening, so that they hear what you have asked them to do.

Remember, if you can, to use choices to encourage your child to do something. If they really are not doing what you have asked them to do then remind them of the house rule and follow the steps you have decided to take when that particular rule is broken.

If you have ADHD yourself you might have to work harder to be consistent and remember what you set as house rules and sanctions. Make sure you do not jump to a more severe sanction than you would have used if you took time to stop and think first.

Reward yourself for each task learned and completed (for example, treat yourself to an evening out with friends or your partner).

Remember you are working hard to help yourself and your child... You deserve a reward!

You might have to be even more organized than other parents and get up earlier to have all the children's lunch boxes ready and all your own preparations done, so that all you have to do in the last hour before you set off is sort out your child with ADHD and your other children in the morning before school and work.

In each step we will outline some tasks for you to do and skills for you to learn, so that you and everyone who looks after your child will be able to find new and more effective ways of dealing with your child's ADHD behaviours.

How Does ADHD Appear in Your Child?

GOAL FOR STEP 1

The goal for Step 1 is really to understand your child's ADHD behaviours. Each child with ADHD is unique and it is important to recognize the behaviours your child needs help with. If you understand the behaviours that result from ADHD you can start to plan how you might intervene. It is important to have the courage to change long-established behaviours and interactions for the benefit of both you and your child.

It may be necessary to change the way you organize your life to make time to change how you interact with your child. *You are going to become your child's guide and trainer.*

Skills overview for Step 1

The skills you will acquire during this step in the programme are:

1. *Making eye contact* while giving your child praise – when they are confident in looking at you, then you will learn how to encourage your child to use eye contact when they are speaking to you and make sure you do the same when you are speaking to them.

2. *Recruiting your child's attention*, how to gain your child's attention before giving instructions.

3. *Listening, and helping your child to listen.*

4. How to start *noticing the good things* your child does and how to praise them so as to *catch the good.*

5. How to become aware that your child copies you (*mirror image*).

6. How to begin to *notice what your child is able to do.*

7. Practising how you and your child *speak to each other showing respect.*

Tasks overview for Step 1

The tasks you will carry out later in this step in the programme are as follows:

- Read about ADHD again to make sure you understand the difficulties your child may be experiencing.

- Discuss all the information you have gathered about why a child with ADHD behaves the way they do with your partner or relative or friend so that you can agree on how to change your approach to your child (with their help and support if possible).

- Practise all the ideas and keep a diary of how events have been and why some strategies worked, and others did not.

- Make a note of your child's ADHD behaviours that are difficult.

- Make a note of your child's ADHD behaviours that are good.

- Write down a list of all the instances of your child's good behaviour (in the diary for good times)!

- Write down all the difficult times you had with your child (in the diary for difficult times).

Initial tasks: Preparing yourself

Make sure you understand about ADHD. Try to think about why your child has the problems they do. This will help you to understand why your child behaves this way. It will also help you to find different ways to get them to do what you want. Read Part I again if you need to. Work on having the courage and energy to change things: this will be good for your child and you.

Remember children with ADHD have difficulty listening and paying attention. They also have difficulty waiting and taking turns. They can also be impulsive, which is why they interrupt so often. This may happen a lot when you are trying to do something you want or need to do, like using the telephone.

This will not be easy and you will have to practise using all the ideas in this book. You may think nothing is changing at first but keep going, *things will get better.*

> Discuss with your partner or a relative or family friend how you are going to work on changing your approach to your child. Enlist their help and support if possible. It is important that all who look after the child work the same way and are consistent.

You need to ask yourself if you and your partner disagree on how to discipline your child. If you are miles apart on the issue you will need to try to discuss why you do not agree. Agree if possible that you will work together over the weeks trying out the ideas and talking together to reach a common way forward.

So try to discuss and talk about the contents of the book at each step and encourage your partner to read and take part in the programme. Listen to yourself when you ask your partner, or a friend, to do something for you. Do you treat your child with the same respect you would use toward your friend or partner. Practise how you want to speak to your child and think through how you are going to speak to them.

Think how you might have to change the way you organize your life to make time to change things with your child. You may need to work on your own organizational skills. We will be asking you to help your child be better organized and think through events before they happen. We will be suggesting to you that you try to anticipate when events and situations might go wrong. This will mean that you will have to be organized as well. You will have to take time to note ways that your child might react so you can work out the pattern of how they behave.

Use this example notepad as a template for keeping your own notes and records about your child's ADHD behaviours and the things they are good at.

We will ask you to keep a diary as you go along so as you can note down how you are doing (example diaries are at the end of the step). This will allow you to see how you are doing but also so to identify all the positive things that your child has done. *Remember you are important as you are going to be your child's guide and trainer, helping them to develop new ways of behaving.*

NOTEPAD

Keep a note of the ADHD characteristics/behaviours you notice in your child here.

I note my child has the following ADHD characteristics/behaviours:

. . . .

. . . .

. . . .

. . . .

. . . .

. . . .

. . . .

. . . .

. . . .

My child is good at:

. . . .

. . . .

. . . .

. . . .

. . . .

. . . .

. . . .

. . . .

. . . .

Skill 1: Making eye contact

Before giving your child instructions it is very important to get your child's attention. Do not shout messages from room to room. Go and find your child.

1. Address them by name.

2. Try to establish eye contact. At first you should only do this for good or positive behaviour or the child will look away, thinking that they are going to be told off.

This is a very simple skill but a very important one. Your child needs to be able to look at you without the fear of being told off, so we ask that you *do not make eye contact when you are telling your child off* but only when you are pleased with them. To encourage eye contact you may need to crouch down and be at your child's eye level. You may need to hold the child's head gently. A tickle under the chin can be a starting point but both hands may need to be used to get the child to look directly at you. Say '[child's name] look at Mummy/Daddy, please' and then say something positive like 'you are really good at eating your dinner today'.

TIPS ON EYE CONTACT

Most children with ADHD are not good at making eye contact. This can be for a number of reasons but one major cause is that they have been told off so many times they have learned to avoid looking you in the eye.

To help your child regain this skill, practise giving them eye contact for positive interactions when they have done something well. They will soon start to look at you more often, and from then on you can start using eye contact for instructions. You are aiming for 10 positives to every 1 instruction initially – this is a high ratio while they learn that giving eye contact is okay again.

Skill 2: Recruiting your child's attention before giving instructions

Once your child is used to looking at you when you are giving them praise then you can use eye contact when you are giving them instructions.

Your child must be in the same room as you. If they are upstairs on the computer or in another room watching TV there is no point shouting a message from room to room. You will have to go to them. Gently address your child. Ask them to look at you and give them your message. If you are successful, and your child responds, thank and praise your child for looking at you.

> **IMPORTANT NOTE**
> Many children with ADHD can concentrate for some time on tasks they enjoy (for example, watching TV or YouTube, playing games on the computer and other non-challenging fun activities).
>
> If you were out to dinner and enjoying yourself, and without notice someone came and whisked you away, you would not be very happy. It is the same with children with ADHD. If your child is one minute engrossed in an activity and suddenly asked to come to dinner or to stop what they are doing and go shopping, without preparation, it is not surprising that they may have a flare-up.

Because of this difficulty with being interrupted, it is important that you take the steps outlined below.

- *Be in the same room as your child.* Shouting at or speaking to your child when they are in a different part of the house is unworkable. It will appear that they have not heard you if you are not in the same room. This is not deliberate on their part. They can 'switch off' if they are enjoying themselves and intrusion into their play or activity will not be noticed. They are still enjoying themselves, unaware that you have become annoyed because they have not responded. *You need to be beside them and gain eye contact to make sure they have heard you.*

- *Give them notice in advance.* Give your child this opportunity to adjust – time to switch off, and time to restart. Just like a computer update, which needs programs to be shut down before it can update, which takes a few minutes, your child with ADHD needs time to change from one task to another. Children who have ADHD need to be cued or signalled into a change of task.

An example of cueing and preparing your child would be to say, 'We are going shopping soon, so you will have to stop playing in ten minutes,' then 'Remember we are going shopping. You will have to stop in eight minutes...in five minutes. Three... In two minutes I will come up and then you must stop your game, turn the computer off or pause the game.' Cueing needs to be done gently but firmly with no room for manoeuvre, so eventually the child gets the hang of it.

Skill 3: Listening and helping your child to listen

Once you have gained your child's attention, make sure they are listening. Tell them what you want them to do *using short sentences* to keep them listening. Tell them one idea at a time.

If your child wants to tell you something, try to stop what you are doing and turn and face them. Make it clear to them that you are listening. If you have to finish what you are doing, ask them to wait. Hold their hand if you can so they know that you are attending to them, and you will really stop what you are doing. Then stop the activity you were involved in as soon as possible and turn to face them so you can listen. This is a visual demonstration of what you will want them to do themselves later (mirror image).

It is useful to repeat what they have said to you so they know you have heard them. Then give an answer. If possible, prolong the conversation, for example by replying with a question so they have to answer.

Skill 4: Notice the good things your child does and praise them: 'Catch the good'

This skill is to help you to start to really 'scope' your child's abilities but focusing on all the good things they do. Most behaviour change happens when people notice what we are doing well and compliment us and then we try to do more of it, or we are pleased that someone has noticed our hard work. Children with ADHD are the same, they work much better when people notice when they are doing things well but they need lots of encouragement to remember to keep doing these things, so 'scope' every good thing they do, make notes and remember to really praise them, so that they do more of these good things.

Try to identify positive features in your child.

Children with ADHD are hard work for any parent or carer, and they are often viewed in a negative way. For some parents it can be very difficult to find anything good about their child. This can lead to a cycle of negativity and parents may have forgotten how to praise their child. They may find that they cannot bring themselves to give praise because they cannot forget the naughty things their child has done at another time. It is important to treat your child as you find them and not to be affected by your residual feelings about incidents that are over and done with.

Try to work towards viewing your child more positively instead of looking at the more negative aspects. Your child and you may well be out of harmony and this may have made discipline problems get bigger. This may cause over-reactions from both of you to every issue.

Start with small nuggets of praise. When your child does something good say 'well done' and at the same time emphasize what they have done so they know what it is you are praising. For example, say 'Well done, Johnny, for tidying your toys up. I'm really pleased with you.' This is known as *capturing the moment of good behaviour*. This is especially important for a child with ADHD as they may well have done something good but then quickly gone on to do something wrong. For example, it is important that a child knows they are being praised for stopping jumping on the chair, not for doing what they did next, which was to snatch their brother's toy car.

Later, aim to use praise to encourage longer periods of acceptable behaviour too, for example 'When you did that [say what it was], it made me so proud [or pleased, happy, delighted, glad etc.].'

Words such as 'good' and 'bad' need to be broadened because they are words that we tend to use excessively and because the child may not really have an understanding of what good and bad really mean. That is why you need to say to your child precisely what they did that you disliked or approved of.

You can also praise using body language, a smile, thumbs up, wink and so forth. Later, written praise can be given if the child understands, such as kisses (xxxx) on notes you write them. Later in the book we will also cover the use of emojis to praise your child.

Skill 5: Be aware that your child copies you: Mirror image

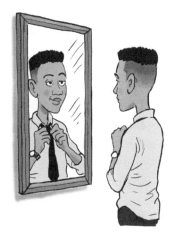

When you are praising, observe your body language. For example, when you say well done do you genuinely mean it or is your body language wrong? Are you smiling or not, are you frowning, looking angry? It is hard if you are depressed or unhappy but it is worth highlighting that if you are going to praise your child, then *try to smile*, even if you do not feel like it. If your child hears you saying 'well done' but you are frowning or looking cross, the child will get a mixed message and doesn't really know what you are trying to say. Remember most children (like adults) look at the eyes for clues to emotion and the meaning of messages.

Modelling behaviour to your child, especially if their learning style is visual, can be a really powerful way to show them how to behave.

Young children copy their parents' actions and so demonstrating how to behave across situations and practising this with them can really help.

Skill 6: Begin to notice what your child is able to do

Start noticing the extent of your child's abilities so you know what you need to work on to change things. For example, your child might be able to concentrate for only three minutes on a game or colouring.

Even though you may think that they should be able to dress themselves, when you watch them you may realize that they are so easily distracted that you may need to be with them to encourage them to stay on task with gentle reminders. Noticing what your child can do or has difficulty with is called *scoping*.

It is important in this step to note how long your child can wait for, how long they can concentrate for and to generally keep note of what your child can do. *Scoping makes you aware of where they are experiencing difficulties and what they will need you to help them with.*

Skill 7: Remember to speak with respect to your child

Talking in a calm factual way helps your child to learn to speak to you with respect. You should speak to your child as you would a friend or colleague so you both learn to interact more positively.

Tasks for Step 1 you need to carry out now

Make sure you understand as much as you can about ADHD and how this affects your child by reading more about it, for instance, why not consider getting hold of some of the resources we list later in the book.

Keep two weekly diaries, one for positives and one for difficult situations

We ask that you keep two diaries: one to write down any difficult situations that have arisen and the other to write down all the things that have gone well. The diaries can be used to see how practising the ideas has gone, and they provide you with the opportunity to review why you think some things have worked and others have not. We have included two diary pages for you to complete, one for good and one for difficult times, at the end of each step in the book. You could make your own diaries if you prefer.

If you are in a partnership share with your partner the things you have noticed your child has difficulty with and the things they are good at. Complete the diaries together if possible. If not, make sure you are working together and support each other in helping your child to learn from you. If you can agree on how to manage your child it provides them with consistency and they know both parents understand their difficulties and are trying to help them.

If you are a sole parent using a trusted relative or friend can be helpful or keeping note in a diary so you can keep track over time of what you are noticing.

Recap and review

What we have covered in Step 1 is reviewed below. Don't just skip this section. Use it as a checklist when you look back at your diaries for the week. How well have you done in achieving the goal? Which skills did you find easy to use and which more difficult? Have you carried out all the tasks?

Goal for Step 1

The goal for Step 1 was to really understand your child's ADHD behaviours. Each child with ADHD is unique and it is important to recognize behaviours your child needs help with. If you now understand the behaviours that are caused because of the ADHD you will be able to start to plan how you might intervene. It is important to have the courage to change things for the benefit of both you and your child.

It may be necessary to change the way you organize your life to make time to change the ways you interact with your child. It is worth repeating – you are on the way to becoming your child's guide and trainer.

Skills summary for Step 1

The skills you acquired in this step were (tick those you have managed to do):

1. I have made eye contact while giving my child praise. As they become confident in looking at me I will then encourage them to use eye contact when they are speaking to me.

2. I have remembered to recruit my child's attention before giving them instructions.

3. I have considered how I listen to my child and how I

demonstrate the importance of listening carefully to my child so they can learn from me (modelling and mirror image).

4. I have noticed all the good things my child does and remembered to praise them so as to 'catch the good'.

5. I am becoming more aware of how my child copies me (mirror image).

6. I have practised speaking to my child showing respect.

The tasks for Step 1 reviewed

- I have read about ADHD again to make sure I understand the difficulties my child may be experiencing.

- I have been discussing all the information I have gathered about why my child with ADHD behaves the way they do with my partner and/or relatives and friends so that we can agree on how to work on changing our approach to my child.

- I have practised all the ideas and written in the diaries how the week has been and why some elements in this step worked and others did not.

- I have made a note of my child's ADHD behaviours that are difficult.

- I have made a note of my child's ADHD behaviours that are good.

- My partner/friend/relative and I have written down all the good things my child did (in the diary for good times).

- My partner/friend/relative and I have written down all the difficult times we have had with our child (in the diary for difficult times).

If you think you understand how your child's ADHD is affecting them and have practised the skills and completed the tasks you can now move on to Step 2. Remember that you can repeat a step at any time if you need to, and each parent can move through the steps at their own pace.

Diary for good days

Day/Date . . . .

Time . . . .

What made it good? . . . .
. . . .
. . . .
. . . .

What did you do? [praise, smile, emoji] . . . .
. . . .
. . . .
. . . .

Did it help your child? . . . .
. . . .
. . . .
. . . .
. . . .

How do you feel now? . . . .
. . . .
. . . .
. . . .

How do you think your child feels now? . . . .
. . . .
. . . .
. . . .
. . . .

Diary for difficult days

Day/Date ....

Time ....

Trigger (what led up to the difficulty) ....
....
....

What happened? ....
....
....

What did you do? ....
....
....

Did it help? ....
....
....

How do you feel now? ....
....
....

How do you think your child feels now? ....
....
....

Looking back would you do anything different? ....
....
....

Strategies to Help Children with ADHD

Skills overview for Step 2

The skills you will acquire during this step in the programme are:

1. How to start using *scaffolding* to see what your child can do.

2. How to identify and use *teachable moments.*

3. How to use *earshotting.*

4. How to adopt a *consistent routine.*

5. How to set clear *behaviour boundaries* and *house rules.*

6. How to use *countdowns* and *delay fading.*

7. Learning to give *clear messages* (remember eye contact).

8. Using short sentences.

9. Using choices.

10. Avoiding confrontations and arguments.

11. Keeping calm.

12. Calming your child.

Things to remember (when changing your approach)

First, it is important to realize that change rarely happens overnight and that it may take a few months to see a significant improvement. We know the skills you adopt will help you to teach your child and improve their skills over time. However, we would expect that you will see change in some things immediately.

Try to ensure that all the adults who look after your child agree how to handle their behaviour and do so in broadly the same way. Consistency is very important. As we have already said it is important for parents to try to accept the child they have. The child's temperament is the way it is and, by adjusting your parenting style, life can become more pleasant for the whole family.

Later in this chapter are some diary pages to help you assess your child's abilities. You can use these to help you see your child's progress over time.

Some parents find some skills easier to adopt than others. If you are having difficulty using a particular skill ask your partner if they are experiencing the same difficulty. If they are you may be able to think of an alternative together which achieves the same goal. *Don't give up, keep trying.* Sometimes it just needs a bit more practice.

Tasks overview for Step 2

The tasks you will carry out later in this step in the programme are as follows:

- Continue to work together with your partner.

- Remember to keep trying skills out over and over again – usually we suggest practising in the home first while you gain confidence.

- Learn to manage behaviour while being realistic about what you can achieve.

- Remember to practise the skills from Step 1, including eye contact, listening and praise.

- Start playing games to help improve your child's attention.

- Play together for at least ten minutes a day.

- Keep a diary for difficult times.

- Keep a diary for good times.

Thinking through how the first step has gone

Have you managed to identify positive things that your child has done and praised them, making sure it was clear what you were praising them for? Looking at the diaries from Step 1 you should have some examples of what went well and what helped to ensure things went well.

Have you made the connection between your child's behaviour and the reasons why he might behave the way he does? Remember, due to their ADHD your child may find it hard to listen and to remember what you have asked them to do. They may start off doing things and then get distracted (very annoying to a parent but understandable for a child who finds it hard to stay on task). We will encourage you to help your child finish something they have started.

Spend time looking at your diaries of both the difficult and the good. See if you can identify triggers for difficult situations.

If you can see a pattern it helps you to avoid repeating difficult events in the future, for example is it a certain time of day or when asked to do a particular thing?

As your child's parent, you are their guide and trainer. We can give you advice and ideas but you will have to carry them out yourself (we hope with the support of a partner or friend).

Skill 1: Scaffolding

Every child has different skills and it would be helpful to take some time to map out what your child can do. As mentioned in Step 1 we call this scoping. Scoping is when you as a parent assess the range of your child's abilities at this moment in time. The *planner* at the end of this week's notes is for you to use to map out what your child can do. Scoping is the first stage of what is called scaffolding.

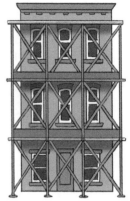

For example, how long can your child concentrate for? We can build on getting them to concentrate for longer. How good are they at listening or coming when you ask them to? Once you have built up an idea of how long they can wait or how well they listen you can build on their abilities and help them to extend their skills.

Knowing how your child is functioning can help you pick the right level of toys or games for them to play with and enables you to judge when to challenge your child to improve their development. This gradually builds up the set of skills which your child can do easily. You then *extend* their skills with tasks that might take a little longer without the child getting cross and losing interest or, just as important, losing their self-esteem.

The stages of scaffolding are:

- *Scoping*: watching your child to see what they are able to do.

- *Mapping their zone of proximal development*: identifying exactly what your child is able to do on their own and how much they could be encouraged to do with you providing the scaffold.

- *Extending*: helping your child to work on a task a little bit harder than they can do on their own.

- *Consolidating*: practising the skills to ensure your child has learned them properly.

We have added a 'Review sheet' for you to complete yourself at the end of this step. It will help you reflect on your child's ability. This sheet will be repeated in Step 6 to enable you to keep a check on your child's progress, and you can design your own too.

Skill 2: Identifying and using teachable moments

Once you suggest a new idea to your child, practise it in different settings. We call that *using the teachable moment.* This means grabbing any opportunity to practise a skill. We are going to suggest games to play with your child that will improve their memory and their attention. You can work on this when you go out on a walk, in the car or in the supermarket, café or pub, or at a friend's house or at Granny's.

Skill 3: Earshotting

Praising in 'earshot' works well. For example, when your child can hear you, say to your partner or friend, ['child's name] did [state what] today and I was so proud of them because they were so [gentle, considerate, kind, affectionate etc.] with [whoever]. Isn't that wonderful.' You can do this on the phone too when your child is in earshot. This skill is really helpful to children who struggle to receive praise as they hear about the good things that they do. Remember, though, to be specific about the praise you are giving.

Skill 4: How to adopt a consistent routine

Provide routine. A child, particularly a child with ADHD, needs to know in advance what is going to happen each day. If the routine changes, let them know. Plan ahead. Plan around tiredness, sleep, hunger and expected mood changes. Visual planners made with the child can be really helpful for them.

Try not to go shopping when the child is hungry or tired, it will only cause difficulties.

Children with ADHD do not like any change of routine. Plan ahead for the day, give advanced warnings, discuss what you are going to do and reassure your child that it will be okay. On the other hand, *do not tell your child about events that are happening many weeks in advance,* otherwise you will be badgered about 'When? What? Where?' Children with ADHD struggle to understand the passage of time and so time perception can be challenging for them.

Here's an example: 'Tomorrow we are going on a trip, by car, with Daddy. We are going to stop at [place] to have a lovely picnic together. Then we will drive a little bit more and then we will arrive at Grandma's. At Grandma's we will have tea and then you can play with Grandma and Grandpa. Then we will drive back home in the car.'

Scope what your child is capable of coping with remembering. If the above is too much information, give them as much advance knowledge as they can cope with, and then give out more as you go along. It might be that you need to scope the whole trip so you know in advance how long they can cope with being at the grandparents' house before they start to struggle. The idea is to work within their abilities and gradually challenge these over time, building up their tolerance to waiting but also their understanding of time.

Keep a diary and note any difficulties carrying out the above tasks. Talk them over with your partner. It is useful to keep a diary so you can look back and compare notes week by week.

Below we give an example of a plan (again, share only as much as your child can cope with at a time).

Planners using pictures

For some children drawing pictures of the plan of the day works well, especially for children who do not yet have good language skills. You can cut out pictures from magazines to aid this.

A normal day plan might have less on it, but you could have pictures you use every day, for example for breakfast, school and so on. This is especially helpful for children with poor language and those who are unable to read yet.

If your child has problems with unstructured time it is worth putting 'free time' in their planner and then help them to structure their own time using their own ideas.

SATURDAY'S PLAN

8.00 am   Get out of bed

8.15 am   Wash face and clean teeth and get dressed

8.30 am   Eat breakfast

9.00 am   Pack your toys to take to Granny's (remember books and toys)

10.00 am   Arrive at Granny's, have a drink and PLAY

12.00 pm   Lunch with Granny and Grandpa

1.00 pm   Go for a walk

2.30 pm   Have a drink and snack with Granny and play games

4.00 pm   Go home in the car

5.00 pm   Play with the grown-ups or watch TV before tea

6.00 pm   Eat tea

7.00 pm   Have a bath, clean teeth and go to the toilet

7.30 pm   Bedtime and story

7.45 pm   Lights out, time to sleep

Skill 5: Setting clear behaviour boundaries and house rules

Having boundaries means setting limits and rules. Children need boundaries, otherwise they do not feel safe. Sometimes boundaries or limits are not clear. We tend to forget to say 'This is what I/we expect of you.' In the case of a strong willed child we tend to

- give in to the child

- be too busy or tired to get them to obey requests

- make excuses, such as 'it's a stage they are going through'.

Children often do not actually know if their behaviour is acceptable or not, unless you tell them. Children will test their parents daily. They want to see if you have moved the goal posts and if they can really trust you. If you keep moving the limits or goal posts or don't stick to the rules you have made your child may become anxious and frightened, and their behaviour frequently reflects this. This is even more likely to happen to children with ADHD. This is because they tend to make lots of demands each day. So as their parents you need to have even more understanding, insight, energy, patience, maturity and creativity than other parents.

We are not talking here about 'obey or else' situations, which will cause the child to behave out of fear rather than respect. You need to be warm, gentle and clear to enable your child to respect you. This also helps the child to respect authority from other people such as playgroup leaders and school teachers. Again, setting an example in the family is important, for example, if parents are rude with friends or relatives, this is what the child learns to imitate (another example of *mirror image*).

House rules

This week decide on a rule you are going to work on and praise the child when they follow that rule. Start with something simple like reminding them that they have to come when called, for example when it is lunch time, and then praise your child when they come when asked to do so. (You can still use countdowns to help them.)

You want to start helping them to understand that when they do what they are asked to do you will praise them and be pleased with them.

Discuss with your partner which rules are important, and which are not. Decide which ones you are going to work on first. Pick only one or two, not more than three, to focus on at a time. Write them down. Make sure everyone in the house agrees what they are going to be and sticks to them. *Remember to make sure that your child is praised for keeping the rules.* Work out a system for accompanying praise with a concrete reward, for example an extra story or more time to watch a favourite program.

It is important that everyone sticks to the rules and that if the rules are broken that everyone has to follow the consequences that have been agreed. It may seem strange but if the parent breaks a rule they should demonstrate to the child how they are following the consequence for breaking that rule, for example, 'Mummy said something unkind to Daddy and so she has to go to the step to think about what she said and how to say sorry.' Demonstration of ownership of our actions and how to apologize is an important part of life to learn.

Remember, though, that first of all you have to get your child's attention. Make sure they have listened and understood what you have asked them to do. Always remember to *catch the good*: when your child has done something good *praise* them. If you think your child will understand you can start working out rewards for good behaviour, once you have established a pattern of praising their good behaviour, for example stickers or extra time playing.

TIP ON THE IMPORTANCE OF PRAISE

Praise your child whenever you can.

Look pleased to see them when you pick them up from school, they may have had a hard day. Remember children often act out what they see! You smile, they smile!

Skill 6: Using countdowns and delay fading

This skill targets time perception as this can be difficult for the child with ADHD to learn.

Reminders such as clocks, timers and warnings are ways of letting your child know that something is going to happen very soon (for example bedtime or going to the shops). All children benefit from having reminders, as they are a clue to jog their memory. Reminders are also less likely to prompt a refusal or a power struggle than an outright command. Children with ADHD have much more difficulty managing time than those without ADHD. Therefore it is very important that these children practise time management. These are techniques that have to be learned.

Use visual clues for recognition of time with your child. For example, show, explain and say 'When the big hand is on [show child] we are going to... .' We are not expecting you to teach a young child how to tell the time but even small children can manage to see the big hand on a clock has moved by five minutes.

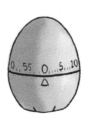
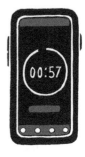

Buzzers, timers (like an egg timer) and alarms are also useful aids to remind the child about time.

TIPS ON THE USE OF TIMERS

Timers can be used in all sorts of ways:

- ▶ to help remind the child of a change in situation ('When the timer goes off we will leave Granny's to go home')

- ▶ to start a new task ('It's now time to clean your teeth')

- ▶ to have 'calm down' time (either for the child or yourself)

- ▶ to signal the start and end of a period of 'fun time'.

Countdowns and warnings

Countdowns, when you tell your child 'We are leaving in ten minutes', 'We are leaving in five minutes' and so on, give the child time to prepare to finish their task compared to a sudden 'We are going now' without a warning, which would inevitably cause a scene. Remember to keep warning the child with time cues. When it comes to the last two minutes: 'I will be up in two minutes and you will need to stop playing, save your game'. Make sure your child knows that they will have to stop and do not allow them to try to prolong the game. They will gradually get the message that stopping time is stopping time. You can also get your child to say back to you the time when you have to leave to check if they are retaining what you have said.

Teach your child to cope with waiting for something they want. We call this *delay fading*. For example, your child wants a biscuit. Lunch is going to be in ten minutes. You answer 'Lunch is in ten minutes – you can have a biscuit after lunch' (*note that you avoid the word 'no'*). Then say 'Let's see what you can do to make waiting for lunch easier. Do you want to do a drawing or some colouring or build me a Lego car?'

Of course what is really important is that you also pay attention to time. If you say to your child that you will be ready in a minute, is your minute really a minute or actually five or ten minutes? Think about what message you want to give your child about keeping to time.

Always keep your warnings and countdowns clear and brief.

Waiting for children with ADHD is almost painful for them, so helping them to learn to tolerate waiting is important. They are probably never going to like doing it, but to be 'waiting neutral' can really help to prevent outbursts. So scope how long they can wait and gradually build up their tolerance.

Skill 7: Giving clear messages (remember to use eye contact)

There is no point in asking your child to do things which are too complicated. Keep your sentences and commands short. *Keep it simple* (KIS) with one idea per sentence. Do not give your child more than one command at a time until you are sure they can manage to remember more than one (an example of *scoping*).

When you want your child to do something, first make sure you have eye contact and your child is listening. Speak in a clear voice, indicating that you expect them to do what you ask them to do. This does not mean an angry voice, just a voice that is firm (like when a bus driver says 'move along the bus' or 'take your seats'). When you want something done, give commands not questions. If you say 'Will you tidy up now?' your child can always answer 'No'. Instead say 'Let's tidy up now, please.'

Skill 8: Using short sentences

Remember, *keep it simple* (KIS) – use short sentences.

Children with ADHD have poor short-term memories. This means they cannot remember long or detailed tasks.

Practise a one sentence rule, with sentences of no more than three to four words, and perhaps ask your child to repeat it back to you when you've said it. This helps them to remember.

Skill 9: Using choices

When you do give choices, give only two choices. This will make it easier for your child to make up their mind and reduces the opportunity for them to say no. *Always make sure that the child has heard the message and understands.* Ask the child to repeat the message back to you.

For example, 'Do you want cheese or ham for lunch?' If your child takes a long time to make up their mind or they are unsure, say 'Are you able to choose today or shall I choose for you? I can see this is difficult for you today.'

You should be aware that in a group situation if all the other children choose something and your child opts for something different your child may later not be happy with their choice. If in doubt say 'Everyone else is having a [item], do you want the same or not?'

TIP ON GIVING TWO CHOICES

Give limited choices, for example 'Do you want a tuna or an egg sandwich?' Remember the child's short-term memory problem and impulsivity, so ask them to repeat what it was they want.

Other examples are 'Do you want me to help you with your coat or are you going to do it yourself?' 'Would you like me to help you clean your teeth or are you going to do them on your own tonight?'

These strategies should lessen the chance of your child replying 'No'.

Skill 10: Avoiding confrontations and arguments

Young children often say 'No'. This is part of normal development, because they are learning to develop a sense of self. They try to discover what power they have. However, they need to learn how to give and take. Try to remember that this challenging behaviour is normal and that you must not feel threatened by it. You, the parent, must try to recognize that after a while the whole argument and confrontation becomes a game. You need to recognize this quickly and ask yourself what is happening, so you can avoid rows. You know that arguments won't achieve the outcome that you want to.

It takes two to argue. You as the parent have to be adult about the situation and say something like 'I have said [avoiding the word *no*] *yes*, you can have a biscuit after your lunch. I am not talking about it now.' You should then walk away. Don't keep the argument going even if your child tries to.

The combination of an upset child and a parent with a short fuse can often mean that major conflicts happen. Many parents with a hyperactive child feel they have tried everything and nothing works. In desperation they may use shouting type behaviour themselves.

Skill 11: Keeping calm

One of the key skills that parents have to learn is *keeping calm*. If you shout, your child also shouts when they are angry and *mirrors your behaviour.* Children copy what they see going on around them and if adults shout at each other when cross your child will do the same when they are frustrated or angry.

Keeping calm is something you have to learn and work at. So practise. Practise and discuss alternatives to shouting with your partner or friend.

One of the techniques that we have found works well is to practise bringing an *imaginary Perspex screen* in front of you (like the shields that police use when they go into riots). You can give yourself a cue to 'bring it down' by rubbing your ear, for example. When you imagine that it is in place you then say to yourself that no negative emotions can reach you. Practise doing this when you feel you are getting angry or anxious. Take a deep breath. If you practise it so that the screen comes down immediately you feel you are getting angry/anxious you can stay calm behind it and deal with your small child more calmly because their crossness 'will not reach you' but you can still 'see out'.

Most parents want to explain to their child why it is so important that they do what they have been asked to. This is fine, but not at the time of crisis.

1. First remove the danger.

2. Let everybody calm down.

3. Only when everyone is calm explain the reasons.

Keep the explanation short and concise – remember the child's short-term memory problems. Do not do the explaining hours later, otherwise the child will have forgotten about the incident.

If the child is in a *dangerous position, always try and stay calm.* Many children have fallen or had severe accidents when someone has screamed and shouted at them. This is difficult because it tends to go against our instincts. Practising calm instructions in a safe environment helps you not to shout in difficult circumstances.

Try to stay calm, try to soften your voice. The child will have to come down to your emotional level to receive your attention.

Here's an example: If you are returning something to a shop, you may be going in ready to have a 'verbal fight' about it. The shopkeeper says calmly 'Yes, Madam. I will refund your money.' This defuses the situation. Try the same technique with your child. Stay calm, the situation could be easily defused if you do not respond by shouting. So *calmly does it*. Give your message in a calm voice and use a respectful tone.

Parents may not like their child having the last word but unless this is a big problem (it is part of normal development, part of developing independence) learn to walk away and not let it irritate you. Remind yourself it takes two to have an argument; one person has to be adult about it and walk away.

Write down what really irritates you and which behaviours can be ignored. For example, whining can be ignored (although it can be very annoying) but some behaviours cannot be ignored, such as hitting, biting and kicking.

Skill 12: Calming your child

If you have an argument with your child they may have a meltdown because they are frustrated, emotionally overloaded, tired, bored, hungry or overstimulated. Meltdowns will be discussed in more detail later.

You cannot ignore the meltdown because through it your child is saying, 'Do something! I am out of control.' By offering to help the child out of a difficult situation you can help to build authority and trust and convey that you are in charge of the situation.

Say calmly 'I can see you are upset. When you are calm we can be friends' or 'then we can have a cuddle'. Try to say this only once. (This acknowledges and names what they are feeling as well as saying you are there and you can talk when we are calm.)

Do not make the message too long. Do not ask why they did

what they did and so on. Ask questions like this only when things are calm. During a meltdown:

- your child is not listening

- your child does not know rational answers anyway (their ability to communicate rationally during a meltdown is impaired)

- you are wasting your breath and energy.

TIPS ON KEEPING YOU AND YOUR CHILD CALM

► Make sure consequences are short and realistic. If possible negotiate these with the child.

► It is better to explain that a rule has been broken and why a consequence has been enforced than to shout.

► Keeping calm is one of the most difficult things to do, but probably the most important.

► Separate the child's behaviour from the child, for instance say 'I love you, but I don't like it when you do...'

► Don't threaten unless you mean to carry through your threat.

► Don't use sarcasm: children with ADHD don't understand it.

Task: Using play to help your child's attention and concentration
Games to help improve memory

Children with ADHD often have problems with attention, concentration, memory, taking turns and losing at games. As a result of this they often find playing very difficult. In the first instance we want the play to be aimed towards your child succeeding, so it is important to prepare before you start to play. Your aim is to help them win by using smaller numbers of cards that you know contain pairs. Over time you should make this more difficult but at first you just want them to enjoy the game and want to play it more.

These games will help your child's working memory. Try to play these games with your child for at least ten minutes a day.

Snap

This game is useful for teaching your child to (1) attend, (2) concentrate, (3) improve their memory, (4) take turns and (5) learn to cope with losing.

The beauty of this game is that as it is a very quick game to play and finish the child knows that a new game will follow in close succession.

Divide up a pack of cards, shuffle them, so that the cards go out of order, then sit facing each other. One by one take turns to turn over the cards placing them in the middle of the table. The first one to spot a pair (a similar card turned up by their partner to the one they have turned up) and shout out 'snap' gets the whole pack in the middle. The game continues until one player has collected the whole pack. Then the next game begins according to the same rules. It is useful to put a time limit on the length of play.

You might want to start playing with only a few cards to at first. If that is the case make sure you have enough matching pairs in the ones you do play with otherwise you and your child will get bored quickly!

Make sure everyone who is playing is playing to the same rules.

You could keep a running tally or work out the winner each time you play.

It does not matter if your child looks at their card at first before laying it down, it is more important for them to feel confident in matching the cards. It is important to help your child win most of the time. You can make it more difficult later on.

TIP: THE IMPORTANCE OF PLAYING TOGETHER

Children with ADHD have problems concentrating. They often miss out on learning through play.

Play games with your child as often as possible (for at least ten minutes each day). Don't make these competitive games but just have a fun time. They can be indoor or outdoor games, whichever you enjoy together.

By doing this you will also help your child learn to play with their friends.

The tasks for Step 2

The tasks in this step have been embedded in the skills. You also need to remember to work together with your partner, family or friends to provide consistency of approach for your child. If possible use the skills from Steps 1 and 2 both at home and outside the home, but in a familiar place, though it is important to practise them as much as possible at home first to give you confidence in using them.

Discuss with your partner whether he or she could play Snap to improve your child's attention. Consider when it is best to play with your child and how to take turns with this. Find ten minutes each day to do this.

Write your diaries for this step, one for difficult times and one for positive times. As in Step 1 these diaries can be used to identify triggers that may lead to a difficult situation (difficult times diary) and those situations which were good and what made them so good (positive times diary).

Recap and review
Goal for Step 1

The goal for Step 2 was to build on Step 1 by understanding your child's ADHD so you can apply the skills described based on your assessment of your child's difficulties. It was about tailoring the strategies to your child's difficulties in your role as your child's trainer.

Skills summary for Step 2

The skills we covered were: (tick those you have managed to do)

1. I have started to use scaffolding and have scoped what my child can do.

2. I have used teachable moments (you can add where and when here).

3. I have used earshotting.

4. I have established a consistent and clear routine.

5. I have clear behaviour boundaries and we have agreed and are using the house rules.

6. I am using countdowns with my child and trying to build their tolerance for waiting (delay fading).

7. I am giving clear messages and remember to use eye contact.

8. I am keeping my sentences short and precise.

9. I am giving choices, and usually just two.

10. I am avoiding rows and starting to use negotiation.

11. I am keeping calm.

12. I am helping my child to experience calmness and to remain calm.

The tasks for Step 2 reviewed

The tasks we covered in this step were:

- I am continuing to work together with my partner, friends and relatives.

- I am working hard to remember to keep trying skills out over and over again.

- I am learning to manage challenging behaviour while being realistic about what I can achieve (it is early days in the programme).

- I am remembering to keep practising skills from Step 1, for example eye contact, listening and praise.

- I have started to play games to help improve my child's attention (Snap).

- We are playing together for at least ten minutes a day.

- My partner and I are keeping a diary for difficult times.

- My partner and I are keeping a diary for positive times.

Assessing your child's abilities

We would like you to sit with your child and watch them with either a jigsaw or pack of cards. If you are using a jigsaw choose one with a small number of pieces, and if you are using cards choose picture cards and start with just a few cards (see 'Snap' above) and get them to match the cards that are the same.

Use the columns below to assess your child's abilities over the next week. Make notes under the headings.

Review sheet

Date	
What are you playing? e.g. pairs, Snap	
How many cards do you think they can manage?	
Did your child manage these?	
Did they require help?	

Making review notes like this is called *scoping your child's abilities*. We have chosen cards and jigsaws on this occasion for you to practise but scoping can also be done for everyday situations like assessing your child's use of a knife and fork or how long they can wait (see the example of headings for this below). Use your notebook to compose your own review sheets.

Date	
What did your child want?	
Did they have to wait to get this?	
What was their behaviour like while they waited?	
How long did they manage to wait until they received it?	
Did they require help – use of a timer for example?	

Assess what your child can do easily now, and then extend this either by increasing the number of jigsaw pieces or cards, for example, or by increasing the time on the timer that they have to wait for something they want.

Once your child has mastered the new waiting time or the new jigsaw pieces (they need to do this a few times so they have really learned the skill) then you can increase the task again. Always increase the task in small steps, for example one extra jigsaw piece, two extra cards or 30 seconds extra on the timer.

It is important when extending a task that you help your child at first. This enables them to keep trying. If your child becomes upset, go back to a previous task they did easily. The aim is to build their self-esteem and failing to do something a number of times will not help with this. Leave the extended task a couple of days and try again, perhaps in a different way.

Do not be tempted to push your child on too quickly. They need to learn the new skill well, and sometimes this can take time. ADHD children tend to rush things and then forget. Doing something well over and over again will help your child to remember the task. We call this *consolidating*. It is also important to try the new skill out in different situations so that the child does not just associate it with the home, for example (use *teachable moments*) and thus generalizing the task to other settings.

Diary for good days

Day/Date . . . .

Time . . . .

What made it good? . . . .
. . . .
. . . .
. . . .

What did you do? [praise, smile, emoji] . . . .
. . . .
. . . .
. . . .

Did it help your child? . . . .
. . . .
. . . .
. . . .
. . . .

How do you feel now? . . . .
. . . .
. . . .
. . . .

How do you think your child feels now? . . . .
. . . .
. . . .
. . . .
. . . .

Diary for difficult days

Day/Date . . . .

Time . . . .

Trigger (what led up to the difficulty) . . . .
. . . .
. . . .

What happened? . . . .
. . . .
. . . .

What did you do? . . . .
. . . .
. . . .

Did it help? . . . .
. . . .
. . . .

How do you feel now? . . . .
. . . .
. . . .

How do you think your child feels now? . . . .
. . . .
. . . .

Looking back would you do anything different? . . . .
. . . .
. . . .

STEP 3

Helping Your Child's Attention and Concentration through Play

GOAL FOR STEP 3
The goal for Step 3 is to help your child learn to concentrate and pay attention through the use of games and play. Play is how children learn when they are young but remains important throughout our lives.

Skills overview for Step 3
The skills you will practise during this step are:

1. Recognizing the importance of play for the child with ADHD.

2. Learning how to use and build on attention-training play.

3. Encouraging listening skills.

4. Using the words 'we' and 'I'.

5. Discussing emotions and extending your child's language.

6. Giving your child choices.

Tasks overview for Step 3

The tasks you will carry out later in this step are:

- Review the skills from the previous steps.

- Review the tasks from the previous steps.

- Use the diaries to see what went well and what did not, and why this might be.

- Play with your child.

- Remind yourself to praise yourself for how well you are doing.

- Remind yourself how important you are as your child's guide and trainer.

- Reflect on your child's behaviours and how they fit into what you know about ADHD.

- Practise instructions in different situations to increase your child's compliance (willingness to do what they are told when asked).

- Review how your child's play is progressing.

- Continue to keep diaries for difficult and good times.

How have the past two steps gone?

Do you think that you and your child are getting on better? Have you remembered to stop and think about their behaviour and how it might be linked to ADHD? Are you praising yourself and the other adults who look after your child for the hard work you are doing trying to change things? Are you using the diaries to review both good and difficult times?

Remember we want to help your child respect you and learn to do what you have asked them to do. *This means that you have to show them respect also.* Getting them to do what you want is a task you have to learn to negotiate together.

Skill 1: Recognizing the importance of play

This step's focus is on play. Play is especially important for children who have ADHD, as they often miss out on areas of play which are vital to development as they are too busy or their concentration span is too short.

Playing is a good way to learn to have fun together as well as an excellent way of teaching your child to wait their turn, learn to win and lose and learn to improve their ability to concentrate and pay attention.

Children with ADHD have poor concentration and will need encouragement to get them playing. This will be valuable in improving their concentration levels. They need rapidly rewarding games – games that do not take more than a few minutes to set up, otherwise they will have lost interest. They can also have low self-esteem, so it is important they start to see a balance in their achievements – games are a good way of helping with this. Games involving taking turns help children to learn to wait. Why not try some of the following:

- Use *role-play games* – such as using toy cars and a road mat to help with road safety skills.

- Use *Lego* people to help teach life or social skills, such as how we join in games and how to express feelings.

- *Reading stories* and looking at the pictures and individual letters in books will lay down some basic skills for reading, as well as helping your child concentrate. This will help your child prepare for school. Research suggests that many ADHD children may be disadvantaged in their early school years if they have not learned the basic appearance of some letters, shapes and the general construction of simple words. Try to spend some time with books. The local library will be useful; staff often run 'reading together' sessions and other events to encourage young children to develop a fondness for books.

- Reading books together can also be a focus for *developing stories together*: 'What comes next do you think, what will happen to the boy?' 'What is he thinking?' 'Does he feel happy?' 'What makes them happy, what makes them sad?'

Playing with your child helps their development. It develops their curiosity and this in turn helps them learn. When you play with your child use language to describe what is happening. That way your child's language skills increase and their ability to express themselves improves.

Children with ADHD have difficulties with attention, impulsivity and hyperactivity. We mentioned earlier that children with ADHD have an active brain too. Therefore these children may also have difficulties with their short-term memory and thinking. Your child may not be good at listening before they respond, they may interrupt conversations and their use of social language and understanding of situations may be poor.

Joint play with your child will help your child begin to value sitting quietly, listening to stories and conversation, taking turns and valuing other people's points of view.

BASIC TIPS ABOUT PLAY

- Let your child initiate the play, so let them choose which game to play, which book to read.

- Follow their direction – don't lead. Try not to tell your child what to do or take over the game. Don't ask too many questions, this disrupts their concentration as they have to think of an answer. For example, don't say 'What colour is that? or 'What are we making?' all the time.

- Don't devalue aimless play – if it is something that fascinates your child then it is important they know you respect their interests.

- If your child has difficulty with play you should guide them but try not to direct them too much. This should be their time with you, not when you impose your ideas on them.

- Children make up their own rules when playing. Try to go along with this.

Helping to improve your child's behaviour through play

It may seem too simple, but play is a really good way of helping your child learn. Often as parents we do not seem to find the time to play with our children. By playing with them we can also give them the message that we want to spend time with them and enjoy their company. Children so often look delighted when an adult joins with them in play.

Teaching your child to play and take turns and negotiate helps them learn to get on with friends and the rest of the family. Help your child learn to play for longer periods by using language to expand their ideas. Describing what they are doing often helps prolong play and adds to your child's enjoyment. *Play helps children learn to express their feelings rather than having to act them out.*

Children with ADHD often rush through play and as a result don't learn how to play well. Play is very important to children as it helps them learn about all aspects of life, including how to interact with other people and so improve their social skills and make friends.

Play can take many forms, from imaginative play to educational play. It is important that children have the opportunity to benefit from as many types of play as possible. Listed below are some hints and tips on how to encourage your child's play and in turn improve their concentration.

FURTHER TIPS ABOUT PLAY

- ► Follow your child's lead – let them choose what they want to play.

- ► Pace the play at your child's developmental level. Don't expect too much.

- ► Do not compete (you are an adult who has already acquired this skill, they have not).

- ► Engage in role-play and make-believe with your child.

- ► Laugh and have fun.

- ▸ Reward quiet play with your attention.

- ▸ Praise and encourage your child's ideas and creativity; don't criticize or directly tell them what to play.

- ▸ Do not give too much help. Encourage your child's problem solving.

- ▸ Tell your child when you have enjoyed play time with them.

Here are some questions and expressions we have heard from other parents about play:

- Why play with my child?

- What is play?

- Do I have to play?

- I don't know how to play with my child.

- I find it boring.

- I don't have time, it's so time-consuming.

- I am too exhausted to play.

For many parents play is seen as a session of somewhat repetitive, boring and thankless activity. With children with ADHD play may well be an additional effort because we know that these children have more difficulty concentrating. They flit from one activity to another and play sessions may sometimes feel unsatisfactory to everyone.

Below we will explain how play can help you and your child. In time play will become fun.

Why play with your child?
You will learn a lot about your child and yourself during play. Play time gives your child the message 'you are worthwhile' and 'you are a valuable person'. It makes your child feel special. If you are not focusing your attention on your child when you play, however, your child will soon know that you have 'switched off'.

Play, believe it or not, can be therapeutic for parents too. When you have had a few play sessions with your child you will start to enjoy it and may find it relaxing rather than taxing.

Bringing up children is hard work, especially today when everyone leads such demanding lives. We are busy and often tired. We buy toys and games that children can play with alone. Aside from the expense, no toy or game can act as a substitute for the personal attention of a parent or learning how to socialize.

We may have forgotten how to play, we may not have had a good model ourselves as a child, it may be difficult to think of ideas for play (see the ideas below). Therefore joint play feels even more difficult to do. With practice and time you will appreciate that joint play is one of the best investments a parent can make. Through playing together you show early on that you are interested in your child, which will help them develop good self-esteem. It will also teach your child vast amounts about:

- communication
- listening
- concentration, attention and working memory
- problem solving
- coordination
- imitation
- creativity
- following directions
- play skills (with others)
- exploration (recognizing smells, texture – such as hard or soft, or directions left and right)
- bonding: improving your special relationship with your child
- social skills (listening, talking, communication, meaning, negotiations, taking turns, sharing, cooperation, friendship and how to resolve conflict)
- awareness of self, others, nature, animals, music, rhythm

- observation

- thinking skills

- independence

- fun!

Play really does help children with ADHD. If you are not already doing so, playing with your child is going to be very beneficial.

Sitting together watching TV, YouTube or on a games console may be a pleasant time. However, it does not generate much interaction between you and your child. For a child, watching TV or YouTube is a passive experience with limited benefits when it comes to socialization and self-development. By discussing the television programme with your child and asking them what happened, what might happen next, was the little boy scared and so on, you can make it into a more interactive experience. It's also important to be mindful of the time spent on all electronic devices (e.g. your phone) as children learn through observation of those around them how to interact with others and their understanding of how to maintain relationships in later life comes from their experiences as a child. So for your play time put away the phone and really spend good quality time in interactions.

When you begin to play with your child, you may have big ideas about what toys would be best. *Remember to start small and keep play simple.* It is best to try to adapt what you already have around the house. There is no need to go out and spend lots of money; your attention is worth significantly more than any expensive toy. First, do not set yourself up to fail by embarking on a complicated game/ toy or idea. *If the play idea takes time to set up, your child's concentration may have run out before you have everything ready, and you will be left feeling rejected and discouraged from trying again.*

Take the example of *painting.* Any paint work should be done with the quickest paint set, only requiring paint, brush, water, paper, some protective paper for the table and your child's apron. Do not attempt to buy individual colour paints that need mixing and take time to prepare. Consider this at a later stage when your child has begun to have fun from painting and can paint for longer.

Try to encourage your child to concentrate and attend to play by talking to them about what they are doing and making it interesting and thus expanding the play. As they learn to concentrate and attend more to play your child will gain more pleasure from play. They will gradually appreciate that sitting down and playing can be fun and they will want to do more. It is important to make positive comments about the play and not to make any suggestions that what they are doing is not good enough. Don't say 'But that does not look like a dog', which will sound negative to the child. Saying something like 'You have drawn a brown dog' is better. You could even say something like 'Remember we saw dogs last week when we walked down the road and you learned their names.' This expands the conversation, suggesting to the child that it can be fun to draw dogs, that you are interested in what they have done *and* you draw on a past situation and connect their painting with something you did together which, in turn, helps them remember.

Some children do not like playing on their own. Showing your child how to achieve results from play, like building or making up games, by taking an interest in what they are doing and praising them and encouraging them, will expand their possibilities for play and keep them interested.

Play ideas

- painting
- drawing with pencils or crayons
- cutting paper shapes (safety and supervision required at all times)
- painting by number
- Lego
- bricks or building blocks
- cars
- dolls
- books
- glue and making things

- what's in fashion (e.g. Paw Patrol, Bluey, Peppa Pig)
- hobbies (e.g. football, cricket)
- cooking: start simply (remember to do it when you have energy, as the kitchen will have to be cleaned afterwards)
- music, singing and rhythm
- poetry and rhymes
- games – such as board games
- what is in season: make Christmas cards, trimmings, birthday cards, a Valentine card, Easter cards – any items appropriate to events you celebrate in your family and that your child enjoys
- playing in the sandpit
- swimming
- dressing up
- pretend play – e.g. shop, schools, housekeeping, cooking, hospitals
- gardening – e.g. pulling weeds, looking at flowers, watering the plants, planting flowers from seeds

Add other ideas that you have here:

. . . .

. . . .

. . . .

. . . .

. . . .

. . . .

Coming up with play ideas can be difficult but the internet has lots of cheap but fun ideas to do with children. Your local library may also have books on play. School staff may give you some ideas as they are continually making things with the children and could remind you of events coming up of interest. For example, for the different festivities and holidays you can make decorations and cards, at Halloween you can make scary masks.

Other family members may also be asked about any tips on play. Having a list of play ideas nearby (for you) can help, especially when you are feeling tired and cannot think of a play idea. You could add your own ideas when you see or think of something that would be helpful.

You will notice that we haven't suggested electronic games, this is because we want you to encourage your child's skills at interacting with others. Children with ADHD can struggle with their interactions with their peer group and so they need to practise these skills in order to know what it is like to wait, take turns, watch others create different play ideas and tolerate this. Online gaming is distant and so the immediate feedback to social cues is lost – the child often won't recognize their friend's emotions (apart from shouting) when they lose a game. Online or computer games also give a lot of visual instant rewards to keep them playing, which for the ADHD child becomes very addictive. So be wary of allowing your child to spend too much time on them as it can become a problem. Time on the games could be earned and allowed for a set time each day.

Skill 2: Attention-training play

While all play is beneficial towards children's development children with ADHD may have specific difficulties, so the games below have been developed through research for their impact on children's attention and concentration. We have found that children's ability to concentrate and pay attention often increases when they practise these with their parents for ten minutes each day. We have suggested and researched these games is because they are quick, easy and cheap to play. A pack of cards, for example, is not expensive to buy. Cards can be carried in your pocket and played with in and out of the home.

(The play ideas in this book have been specially selected to help improve your child's concentration, attention and listening skills.

You may come across other games yourself which you find work particularly well with your child. If you do, write them in your diary and use them again in the future when choosing games for you and your child to play.)

Games will help your child's *visual memory* (Snap, Pairs and Kim's Game) and some will help their *auditory memory* (I Spy, Simon Says, I Went to Market and I Bought (or I Went to the Zoo and I Saw etc). They also help concentration and attention and listening skills.

Scope your child to decide how many cards you can use for Snap or Pairs, for example, and as they get the hang of it increase the number being used. The games also teach turn taking, are fun, and can be completed with everyone feeling in a win-win situation. As they are over quickly if the child loses, you can play again and tell them that they may win next time. *Remember to keep talking as the game begins to encourage your child to stay interested. Agree on the rules before you start playing (that includes for any adults too!).*

Snap

You started playing this in the second week (Step 2).

This game is useful for teaching your child to concentrate, take turns, work on their visual memory and cope with losing. The beauty of this game is that as it is a very quick game to play, and finish, the child knows that a new game happens quickly.

Pairs

This game helps attention training, listening, taking turns and waiting. This builds on the skills learned from playing Snap. It extends the ability of the child to remember pictures.

Take some cards in pairs (say five pairs to start with); picture ones are best. Place them face down on the floor or a table and scatter them around. The aim is to find the matching pairs. In turn, turn over one then a second card. When you find the matching pair remove it from the floor. If the pair does not match turn the cards back face down in the same place on the table or floor. The object is to try to remember where on the floor the pairs are. The player with the most pairs wins. Encourage your child to remember where the cards are on the floor. Remember to praise them for waiting their turn and concentrating on the game. Praise them when they find a pair. *Remember this is your child's chance to win, not yours – it is not a competition with your child.*

Play can be developed further by taking opportunities to match pairs or groups of objects when you are out and about, such as cars of the same colour, same make, same size (grabbing teachable moments).

Kim's Game

Put two items on a tray or in a box. Get the child to look at them, and then cover the items up. Then ask your child to remember what was there. Increase the number of items gradually as your child becomes better at it.

This simple but effective game works on listening skills and visual and auditory memory.

I Went to Market

Taking turns, one of you starts off: 'I went to market, and I bought a loaf of bread.' The next person has to say the same sentence, remember the loaf of bread and one other item, then the next person goes through the same list adding their item and so on. This will build up the child's auditory and word memory and help listening skills. You can make it fun by buying funny items.

You can change it to 'I went to the Zoo and I saw an elephant then a giraffe' or 'I went to the park and I saw a swing' and so on.

Games like this one can be played when waiting for buses, on train journeys, at Granny's (teachable moments).

I Spy

This is a useful game to keep children quiet in the car or on a bus journey, or when they are tired on a walk. It helps them to look around them and take an interest. Remember to make it simple at first so your child understands the rules.

So, the parent will say: 'I spy with my little eye, something beginning with D [or something red, or something you can write with].'

Plan the game at the child's level of skill. Then it is the child's turn.

Simon Says

This is a good game to make children learn to wait and listen. When you say 'Simon says walk two steps', the child is allowed to walk but if you just say 'walk two steps', the child stays still. You can vary it with 'Simon says make a funny face' or anything that makes it fun. This game will help your child's auditory memory as well as their listening and attending skills.

Remember when you are playing a game to set a time limit. It is important that you know how long you are playing for so you can concentrate and not think of all the other tasks you must do. Setting a time limit is also important so that the game has a beginning and an ending, and you both keep to it. It is more useful for your child to play for frequent short periods of time than only one long time that ends in tears. *You could use a timer.*

You will notice the examples above are for younger children; for those a bit older, once you understand the reason behind the games in terms of what ADHD difficulty you are targeting, you can choose more age appropriate games (e.g. for older children 'Guess Who' is a good game for visual skills, Jenga is another for learning to wait, concentration and slowing down).

Reviewing your child's progress with play

Once you have played these games a few times with your child you should start using a play review sheet to assess their progress and make sure you are extending their learning appropriately.

The example we give below is in two sections. The first is aimed at play using the specific attention and concentration games we have suggested to you such as Snap, Pairs, I Went to Market. Using the guide below should help you scope your child's abilities over time and keep a check on how they are progressing.

Assess your child's abilities over the next week and note the following:

Review sheet for attention-training games

Date	
What are you playing? e.g. Pairs	
How many cards do you think your child can manage?	
Did your child manage these?	
Did they require help?	

When you have filled in these play review sheets, make your own in your notepad. The review sheet below is for play that your child chooses, including drawing, painting and so on

QUALITY TIME WITH PLAY

Play is a form of quality time. Try to encourage good quality time (stories, games and so on) between you and your child.

What exactly is quality time? Many people believe that quality time must be action-packed time. This is not true. Quality time with your child can be whatever you want it to be. It could be having a cuddle together, reading a book or playing a game together. Just talking, listening or maybe having some quiet time together. Sharing things together, making supper, going out together.

Children need to know that they are loved and wanted and that you are prepared to spend and enjoy spending time with them. *Do not let bad behaviour be the only way that your child gets attention from you.*

Skill 3: Encouraging listening skills

How do you get your child to do what you have asked them to do?

We have discussed helping your child to listen to you so that they can hear what you want them to do. We have talked about how important it is that your child knows that you are pleased with the good behaviour they have shown.

We have talked about how the way you talk to your child and the way you ask them to do something are important. Practise these essential listening skills as much as you can.

Skill 4: 'We' and 'I' and tone of voice

Enthusiasm in your voice is very important, especially when presenting two choices, since you can use it to highlight the choice that you really want them to make. Speak to your child as you would like to be spoken to. How would you, the adult, address a friend, for example? Speak at the level of understanding of the child.

Speak in a socially correct manner. Start by understanding that if you say 'please' and 'thank you' yourself in appropriate situations, the child will follow your example (mirror image again). Remind yourself that respect is taught and children will not know how to express it automatically.

Use 'we' for house rules, such as 'We walk in this house', 'We are gentle with people and animals', 'We sit on the furniture, we do not jump on furniture', 'We shut doors quietly.'

Try, if you can, to use positive house rules rather than negative ones, for example: 'We shut the door quietly', rather than 'Do not bang the door.'

Draw, paint or write the house rules and display them on the wall. This helps you and your child to remember the agreed rules and they can be used when other children visit. The rules should apply to all children in your house.

When you come across a particularly difficult problem with your child's behaviour try to build a strategy around the problem into the house rules. Make sure that it is attainable and not unrealistic. Eventually when you go out visiting, all that you need to say is 'We know the house rules.'

To recap, by using 'we', we:

- protect our child's self-esteem

- take the pressure off them and make it less likely that they will refuse to stick to acceptable behaviour.

For example, 'We do not do [...] here', 'When you are calm we can talk about it.'

Skill 5: Discussing emotions and extending your child's use of language

Children often have difficulty explaining why they are cross. It is important to help them learn to put emotions into words. Children with ADHD often have problems learning to express themselves and have problems with self-regulation.

For example, sometimes children become cross when asked to do something as they often don't know how to do it. Instead of being able to explain that they shout or have a meltdown. Parents can help their child to learn to share their feelings by talking to their child about times when they have not known what to do or have felt frustrated. This should encourage the child to share rather than act out.

Use the 'I' message. For example, 'When you did [...] I felt happy,' 'When you did [...] I felt sad.' Use broad and clear messages avoiding, if possible, the words good and bad, because your child will not understand what behaviour was good or bad. Explain in simple words what the acceptable or unacceptable action was. This is particularly important as it also introduces children to the concept of all of us having feelings and we hope that over time it will help your child to be able to express their feelings better.

Skill 6: Choices revisited

Remember to keep choices which avoid a 'no' answer. This takes practice for parents but eventually if you do practise it will become automatic. For example, 'Do you want play a game of cards now or later on after lunch?' Change 'no' to 'yes' whenever possible. 'Yes, you can have a [...] after tea', 'Yes, we will go to the park after we...' If you are already carrying out many of the above approaches keep up the good work.

Tasks for Step 3

Take some time to review the skills and tasks from the previous steps. How are these going? Are you using the diaries to review difficult and positive times?

Remember to put aside time to play with your child. Ten minutes each day helps. You can use the timer to signify the start and end of the play time. Are you and your partner working together in your approach to your child to provide them with the consistency they need because of their ADHD characteristics? Remember to praise yourself mentally when you handle a situation well. If you feel confident with a skill in the home start to try it in different situations.

Remember to keep using the diaries.

YOUR OWN MEMORIES OF CHILDHOOD AND BEING PARENTED

We know that parenting a child with difficulties is extremely hard work and that it may bring out memories and flash-backs from your own childhood. How your parents used to discipline you, and how you remember this, could bring back unpleasant or disturbing memories for you.

If it happens you may want to discuss this with someone. Your health visitor or doctor may be able to advise you about whom to contact if you ask them. Don't try to carry on with-out help if you are finding this aspect troubling.

It is essential to work on building your own confidence in your ability to instil a balance of clear boundaries for your child as well as having fun together. Many parents when man-aging a child with ADHD may have low self-esteem. You may have lost your confidence, as other people keep commenting that your child's difficult behaviour is your fault, making you feel inadequate. Understand that this is not the case – your child needs a different sort of parenting to respond and learn from you. Try and choose someone you trust to help you. It could be a partner, friend, parent or health professional.

Recap and review
Goal for Step 3
The goal for Step 3 was to help your child learn to concentrate and pay attention using games.

Skills summary for Step 3
The skills I have practised in this step are: (tick all that you have done)

1. I have joined my child while they played as I understand the importance of playing with my child regularly.

2. I have started doing the attention-training play with them and scoping what they can do.

3. I am listening to them and encouraging them to listen carefully to me.

4. I am using the words 'we' and 'I'.

5. I am expressing and discussing emotions and extending descriptive language when playing.

6. I am continuing to use choices.

Tasks summary for Step 3

The tasks I have practised are:

- I have reviewed the skills from the previous steps.

- I have reviewed the tasks from the previous steps.

- I am using the diaries to see what went well and what did not, and why this might be.

- I am playing with my child.

- I am remembering to praise myself and my partner/friends and relatives for how well we are all doing.

- I am reminding myself how important I am as my child's guide and trainer.

- I spend time reflecting on my child's behaviour and how it fits into what I know about ADHD.

- I am practising more situations to increase my child's compliance (their willingness to do what they are told without a fuss).

- I am continuing to keep diaries for difficult and good times.

You have now completed the first three steps in the programme – well done. There is a lot of information in each of the steps. You should be gaining confidence as you go through each step. Remember children will challenge any change in your behaviour as parents. Stick with it – it does help in the end.

Diary for good days

Day/Date . . . .

Time . . . .

What made it good? . . . .
. . . .
. . . .
. . . .

What did you do? [praise, smile, emoji] . . . .
. . . .
. . . .
. . . .

Did it help your child? . . . .
. . . .
. . . .
. . . .
. . . .

How do you feel now? . . . .
. . . .
. . . .
. . . .

How do you think your child feels now? . . . .
. . . .
. . . .
. . . .
. . . .

Diary for difficult days

Day/Date . . . .

Time . . . .

Trigger (what led up to the difficulty) . . . .
. . . .
. . . .

What happened? . . . .
. . . .
. . . .

What did you do? . . . .
. . . .
. . . .

Did it help? . . . .
. . . .
. . . .

How do you feel now? . . . .
. . . .
. . . .

How do you think your child feels now? . . . .
. . . .
. . . .

Looking back would you do anything different? . . . .
. . . .
. . . .

STEP 4

Improving Your Child's Communication

GOAL FOR STEP 4

The goal for Step 4 is all about helping your child to manage their emotions – this is a skill that can take the child with ADHD a while to learn, and they will need help to learn it. There are several steps needed to help your child with their communication to enable them to express their feelings rather than act them out and learn to manage their behaviour.

Skills overview for Step 4

The skills you will acquire during this step are:

1. Expanding your child's language through play.

2. Working on voice (e.g. volume and tone).

3. Setting clear goals and expectations.

4. Anticipation.

5. How to deal with meltdowns and using distraction techniques.

6. Using the concept of quiet time.

7. Using time out.

8. Cueing your child to tasks and changes of task (Step 2).

9. Coping with delay.

10. Talking about and showing feelings.

Tasks overview for Step 4

The tasks you will carry out in this step in the programme are:

- Review your progress and difficulties from Steps 1–3.

- Remember your role as guide and trainer.

- Recall how important you are as a positive role model for your child.

- Find opportunities for play (quality time).

- Find more teachable moments.

Skill 1: Expanding your child's language through play

Try to put aside time each day to play the games we suggested in Step 3 and enjoy your time together in other ways, such as reading stories, painting, going for walks – whatever you and your child find to do that works for the pair of you. Remember if you talk to your child while you are playing, and praise and encourage them, you will be helping them to feel good about themselves. By using descriptive comments and explanations to extend play you are encouraging them to keep playing and get something out of it.

For example, during your child's bath time when you may be playing with toy ducks you might say 'Do you remember when we fed the ducks?' or 'We saw ducks when we were with Granny' – whatever is appropriate. By using language, you keep the child interested in carrying on playing, as the play has additional meaning.

Skill 2: Working on tone of voice

In the last step we discussed using 'I' statements. The tone of voice you use will also enable your child to understand what you mean. A firm tone of voice highlights that you mean what you say. Praise and a positive tone of voice will give the impression to your child that you are proud of them and their behaviour.

We have talked about using language and the 'I' and 'we' words but how you say things is also very important. Children often pick up more from your tone of voice than what you are saying. Below are some more thoughts on tone of voice.

1. Your voice should remain as calm as possible in difficult situations.

2. Remember to smile when saying something positive; remember to also smile with your eyes. Children look into eyes and if the expression in your eyes does not match the one on the rest of your face your child may not know whether you are happy with them.

3. Your child will watch you and your expressions – check them out yourself in a mirror. What do you look like when you're happy, sad or angry? Does your child look similar when they are happy, sad or angry? Is this how you want them to feel and act?

4. Try to end the day on a positive note. Spend time reminding your child all the good things they have done that day. If they can, get them to tell you the good things they have done too. This helps them to reinforce the good and encourage more of the same behaviour.

Skill 3: Setting clear goals and expectations

A positive targeted approach to rules and expected behaviour will give your child a clear message that you expect them to do what you ask them to do. It is very important to set rules and tasks for them that they will be able to achieve. Try to work out what they can do and set realistic goals. Remember to try to see this as a win–win situation for both you and your child.

If you have observed that your child can sit and play for five minutes, praise them for doing that. Then next time expect them to sit for six minutes and then praise them for doing so. If you know your child can manage to put on their pants and vest without a prompt, praise them for that, and then ask them to put on their shirt too before you come back and then praise them for what they have achieved. If your child can manage to wait for their turn to speak for half a minute, praise them, and then next time help them to wait for one whole minute. *In this way, we are helping you to encourage your child to build up their skills and their ability to solve problems for themselves.*

Just as you have 'scoped' their waiting abilities now start to scope your child's emotional regulation:

- How long do meltdowns last?

- What soothes them?

- What do you notice about their body language?

- Are they aware of any changes in their moods etc?

Skill 4: Anticipation

It is not always easy to predict when things may be difficult, but understanding how your child views the world can help you anticipate situations which they may find difficult. Sometimes using the diaries can help you identify triggers. Many parents notice that their child's behaviour is often worse when they are tired or hungry. It may be easier to lower your expectations of your child at these times, ignoring minor misbehaviour.

If you know your child can usually manage five minutes of play before getting cross or wanting to 'borrow' their brother's toys, then watch and encourage them for playing well for that length of time. If you then see they are about to want their brother's toys, discuss with them how they could negotiate that, or use language to help them play longer with the toys they are already playing with, for example by describing what they are doing or what could happen next.

If your child is about to lose their temper, use some distraction techniques (see Skill 5). Note which one seems to work best with your child.

If your child has problems playing with others it is important that you try to be in the same room with them so you can intervene early. By doing this you will gradually teach your child the art of negotiation so that they will learn to control their temper. As they acquire this skill they will get better at playing independently with their friends. As you become more attuned to your child you will begin to recognize when they are likely to have a meltdown, and you will gradually be able to manage these situations with quiet time (discussed later).

Skill 5: Meltdowns and distraction techniques

If possible, intervene before a meltdown happens. Work out what causes the meltdown and when you see it happening, quickly distract the child with something else. For example, your child is about to have a major wobbly because their younger brother has taken their toy, so you intervene before they do. Have a list of strategies in the back of your mind that could be used for distraction (practise them or write them down).

Use your voice appropriately. Make your tone exciting, signalling enthusiasm in the words that you are using to distract. Make what you are suggesting fun and hard for the child to say 'no' to.

For example, say 'I know that it is not fair that [...] has taken your toy'

'but let's play with this car' or

'Here is some more Lego' or

'I will make sure you both have enough crayons to play with' or

'Wow, look at [...], is it a bird, I wonder what colour it is? Can you see it and then tell me?' (to help distract them) or

'You can draw beautiful pictures. Shall I help you to get...'

Distraction works really well with younger children.

With older children using humour can sometimes help relieve tension but you may need to practise this and make sure it is joint humour, so something your child will find funny too.

Skill 6: Quiet time

Quiet time is a technique to help your child learn to self-regulate their behaviour. This means that over time your child will learn when they are likely to get into trouble or difficulty and give themselves time to calm down.

In the first instance we ask that you use the diaries to identify triggers for difficult situations, for example your child may be able to play with a friend for 15 minutes without any difficulties, but if you leave them for longer they start to argue. If you see signs that your child is getting wound up, ask them at about 12 minutes to come to the 'quiet time mat'. On the mat are some quiet toys. Tell them they can play with them until they have calmed down and then they can return to playing with their friend. You should stay with them next to their mat – *this is not a punishment*. The quiet place should be viewed as a positive zone to give them and you time to calm and to stop situations escalating out of control.

You and your child should discuss when you will use quiet time. For example, use it if you think that your child is about to lose their temper, or if it is clear that a game is getting too noisy and it will end in a fight if not stopped. Quiet time is ideal if your child when playing a game starts thinking that it is 'not fair' and cannot continue without getting into a temper. *Remember it is important to try to help your child reach a stage when they begin to recognize the need for a period of quiet time themselves.*

How to use quiet time or talk your child down

If you can see that your child is about to lose their temper and get cross, withdraw with them to a place that you have already discussed, a step or a quiet place or a mat, something that is easily transportable or transferable to different settings. *Talk quietly to your child* – calm them before something happens. This provides a 'thinking space' that can lower the child's senses if they feel overwhelmed. Sometimes you can use recollected films you have enjoyed for the child to imagine while they are in a quiet place so they can visualize a happy, tranquil scene to calm themselves down. Use the same techniques that you would use yourself, such as breathing slowly and deeply and counting to ten. Your child can be allowed to take toys with them – playing quietly will help. The purpose is for your child to become calm and gradually begin to recognize in themselves the signs that they are getting cross. Later, when calm, outside their quiet space you can talk to them about what they felt and what had started to frustrate them. They may at this point be able to think with you what they might be able to do differently if it happens again, for example, sharing toys, using language to negotiate sharing.

Some children respond to having something tangible to signify their calm down place. A *mat* (a small piece of carpet, e.g. a carpet square from a carpet shop or even a square of material) is useful if needed, as it can be taken to Granny's or used in playgroup and school. The mat needs to be introduced prior to using it for quiet time, so the child understands what is expected and that it is not a punishment. It is a *magic/space carpet for using for quiet time.*

A parent can also use quiet time for space for themselves when they think events may become fraught and they need time away from their child. (Make sure your child is safe, or another adult is available to look after them.) Quiet time, then, can be used as a modelling example from parent to child. You could say 'Do you remember when mummy was cross, she went outside to sit on the step to calm down?' This will help your child learn by example. It is also helpful for you to discuss when your own quiet time might be used with your child so they know when you are likely to need space.

With an older child you can say 'I think we need a period of quiet time. We can sit together and read or draw/colour/play with toys' while expressing it is good to have time together to calm ourselves. If they don't want you to sit with them you can suggest 'You sit there and I will sit over here and we can chat more when we are calm.'

You can use the house rules to reinforce calm down time (e.g. the house rule might be that we play nicely together and your con-sequence could be to have some quiet time apart with lots of praise for using quiet time) so they know this isn't a punishment but a time to learn to calm themselves with your help.

If the behaviour deteriorates or is unacceptable, for example they have hit their sister or brother, you then might need to use 'time out'.

Skill 7: Time out

Time out is a more extreme measure than quiet time and should only be used as a last resort when distraction, quiet time, presenting your child with choices and other strategies have not worked, and the child's behaviour is unacceptable. It should be used as little as possible, as the aim of this step-by-step programme is to help the child understand, express and learn to control their behaviour. Time out can however be useful in setting firm boundaries around totally unacceptable behaviour such as hitting others. You and your child should decide beforehand what would merit time out, for example hitting another child or parent, throwing things, becoming destructive. This could be written in the house rules as a reminder alongside more positive rules such as rewards for good behaviour.

How to use time out

If your child's behaviour is such that you need to use time out, you would first warn the child. Say to them that they will have to go to time out if the behaviour does not stop immediately. You can use counting, one... two... three, if this will work for your child. But only use one, two, three if time out is the sanction.

Time out is used when your child has done something that is not acceptable. Use a step or a chair or their room if the child will accept this (some children see being sent to their room as rejection and make such a fuss that it becomes unhelpful). If necessary carry the child to time out if they will not go themselves. Make sure your child knows the situations when time out would be used and where it is going to take place.

The duration of time out should be one minute for each year of your child's age to a maximum of ten minutes. If your child comes out from time out take them back and stay with them if they cannot stay on their own, but with minimal contact and no discussion until the time is up. If your child has a sensitive temperament (see 'Children with ADHD who are also temperamentally sensitive' in Chapter 1) staying on their own is very difficult for them. They may need the reassurance of an adult nearby. It is important however that discussion and interaction should be kept to a minimum at this time.

Time out should be used as a last resort if all the other strategies haven't worked. If it is happening too often you should review your house rules with your child, as it may be that by going back over why things are going wrong you might lessen the need for time out. Some children respond better when parents reinforce house rules and boundaries at the beginning of each day. This sends the message that the parents are in charge and can manage their child's behaviour. If your child responds to frequent repetition and statement of boundaries, as they might just need the reminder, being firm at the beginning of the day may reduce the need for time out.

Sometimes you do need to withdraw your child from a situation as nothing else is working. Sometimes you two need time apart to calm down. If you think you need time apart ask your partner or friend to help. Remember it can take you time to calm down. 'When we are both calm we can have a cuddle and we will talk about what happened.' If you feel that you are getting really cross with your child, it might better for both of you to be in different rooms to calm down.

TIPS ON DEALING WITH MELTDOWNS
Here are some ideas for what to do if they've lost it!

- Keep calm, ignore your child's extreme behaviour if possible (remember to use the *Perspex screen*).

- Do not discuss the incident, if the child is in the throes of an outburst they are not listening or able to listen.

- Give them time to calm down.

- Give yourself time to calm down. *It takes the adult brain 20 minutes of time out to calm down.*

- Discuss what could have been done differently with your child at a later time.

- Remember children can come up with great ideas to prevent a meltdown if asked when all is calm again after an episode, so statements like 'Mummy could see how upset and angry you were. Have you any ideas on how I can help you when you are so upset, as you know I can't let you hit your sister as that's unkind.' This is not to go over what they did but to get them to think about what they could do differently next time they get angry.

With the best will in the world parents can become frustrated and angry too, so it is important to walk away from a situation (making sure your child is safe and calling on others to give you a break) when you know you are not in the best frame of mind to manage your own emotions. All of us get angry at times and how we manage this is important.

Skill 8: Cueing your child into tasks and changes of task

We talked in Step 2 about using countdowns into a change of task or situation. For example, rather than just telling your child it is time to leave for school, remind your child that you have to go out in a few minutes (remembering to cue them down in five minutes, in four minutes, as necessary), then remind them at one minute that they will have to stop playing and get their coat and shoes. This gives your child a chance to prepare for, and accept, a change. *Remember children with ADHD may not like change.*

Keep practising this skill, and gradually practise cueing in less when your child becomes better at making the adjustments for regular daily tasks. Use the technique especially for new situations, or when your child is tired, or you have a series of tasks to do, like a complicated morning with shopping in more than one place or visiting friends. It is always important to cue your child into something you want them to do or something you want them to stop doing. Again, asking your child how they like to be reminded can be helpful: do they like visual prompts, auditory prompts or both, or do they need you to be with them?

Skill 9: Coping with delay

Remember you are aiming for them to be able to tolerate waiting.

Helping your child learn to wait is important as many aspects of everyday life require waiting and many children with ADHD find this difficult. You can start by helping your child learn to wait for lunch or a biscuit, or until you have finished doing something. Increase the time they have to wait for things gradually. We call this *delay fading*, as we saw in Step 2. You can use the timer for this.

It is important for children with ADHD to work on their ability to wait, and to become aware of their difficulties, so ask your child 'How long do you think you can wait for [...] today?' so they set their own targets for waiting. You may have to modify these if you do not think they will manage to wait that long. This is part of the scoping you undertake with your child (see Step 2) as it is important that they succeed and are then praised for being able to wait.

Helping the child learn to wait will improve their ability to wait their turn when playing games and waiting for instructions, thus helping the child improve their relationships with peers and adults. It will also lessen the impulsivity of some children with ADHD so they learn to wait instead of running off or butting into conversations.

Skill 10: Talking about and showing feelings

Listen carefully when your child talks to you.

Encourage your child to tell you how they feel. Notice how they seem to be feeling and say to them when they look happy or sad. Being able to communicate feelings helps the child and stops them from acting out their feelings instead.

It can often help children if you explain what you are feeling and why – not necessarily in detail but enough so they can understand your point of view. Children often blame themselves if parents are in a bad mood – they think they must have done something to cause it, when it may be that you have just received a bill you were not expecting. Explaining to your child helps them to know when you are upset and why. *Remember to do this when you are happy too.*

Continue to keep a diary and note any difficulties carrying out the above skills. Remember to keep a diary for positive times too!

TIPS ON THE IMPORTANCE OF FEELINGS

▶ Help your child to discuss their feelings rather than act them out.

▶ Ask them if they are sad, happy or angry. If you've got it wrong, they will tell you.

▶ If your child learns to tell you their feelings, they are less likely to act them out through their temper.

▶ Acknowledging your child's feelings will help them feel listened to. *Don't be tempted to dismiss their feelings.* They will be real to them, even if you do not think they are accurate. You can help them see positives at another time.

▶ You can give your child ideas to manage their feelings, such as punching a pillow when angry or drawing what has made them sad.

▶ Share your feelings with them too. Find ways of dealing with feelings together.

Children with ADHD are often excellent 'people watchers' – they can tell when someone is anxious or unhappy. What they struggle with is working out why, as they often get into trouble because of their ADHD difficulties. They can assume when a person is upset that they have caused the upset when they might not have done. This can increase their anxiety and difficult behaviour, so it is important to discuss feelings and talk about these so that they know they are not always the cause of an upset.

Tasks for Step 4

Remember to review your progress and difficulties from Steps 1–3. Note those skills and tasks you find easy and those more difficult.

Remember that you are acting as your child's guide and trainer and that you are important as a positive role model for your child. Keep finding opportunities to play with your child using both attention-training games and free play where you play games of their choice – both are important.

Try to gain confidence in using the skills in different situations: practise and practise until you feel confident.

Recap and review
Goal for Step 4

The goal for Step 4 was for you to help your child with their communication skills to enable them to express their feelings and learn to manage their behaviour better.

Skills summary for Step 4

In this step you practised the following skills (tick those that you have managed to do):

1. I have been increasing extending my child's language when we play.

2. I am working on my voice and keeping my voice calm and with an even tone.

3. I have set clear goals and expectations.

4. I am using anticipation to prevent difficult situations.

5. I am practising dealing with meltdowns and using distraction techniques.

6. I am practising using quiet time.

7. I am only using time out for very serious misbehaviour.

8. I am practising how I cue my child into tasks and changes of task.

9. I am helping my child to tolerate waiting.

10. I am naming and talking about feelings.

Tasks summary for Step 4

In this step you carried out the following tasks:

- I have reviewed my progress and difficulties from Steps 1–3.
- I have remembered my role as guide and trainer.
- I am aware of how important I am as a positive role model for my child.
- I have found opportunities for play (quality time).
- I have found teachable moments in all steps of the programme.

Step 4 can be one of the most challenging for parents. Managing your child's difficult behaviour, in a way that they can learn to eventually manage themselves, is hard and it can take a long time, sometimes years. Persevere. Helping your child to learn to regulate their own responses is an extremely important skill for children with ADHD. If this skill is established early on in childhood it will help your child considerably in their teenage years when children tend to be able to communicate less because of the changes that are happening in their brain and bodies. Ensuring that communication between you and your child is as positive and effective as it can be before they become a teenager helps both of you learn to negotiate early on and can prevent many difficult situations in the future.

QUALITY TIME IN GENERAL

Quality time is important for parents and children. By quality time we mean time that parents and children spend doing something that both want to do and that is fun. Reading stories together, playing games, painting, cooking – anything that is quiet and fun and not demanding. Parents should try, if possible, to build some time during each day for this – it does not have to be for long. Even ten minutes when the child feels that their parent is devoting their time to them works well.

Diary for good days

Day/Date . . . .

Time . . . .

What made it good? . . . .
. . . .
. . . .
. . . .

What did you do? [praise, smile, emoji] . . . .
. . . .
. . . .
. . . .

Did it help your child? . . . .
. . . .
. . . .
. . . .
. . . .

How do you feel now? . . . .
. . . .
. . . .
. . . .

How do you think your child feels now? . . . .
. . . .
. . . .
. . . .
. . . .

Diary for difficult days

Day/Date ....

Time ....

Trigger (what led up to the difficulty) ....
....
....

What happened? ....
....
....

What did you do? ....
....
....

Did it help? ....
....
....

How do you feel now? ....
....
....

How do you think your child feels now? ....
....
....

Looking back would you do anything different? ....
....
....

Managing Your ADHD Child Outside the Home

Skills overview for Step 5

The skills you will practise during Step 5 of the programme are:

1. Listening, sharing feelings, mutual respect and negotiations.

2. Extending the use of timers.

3. Calming your child outside the home.

4. Doing more on 'earshotting' – showing others your child's good points.

5. Repetition of instructions.

6. Using house rules in the outside world.

7. Using rewards.

8. Using teachable moments in depth.

9. Using Social Stories.

10. Using mindfulness.

11. Recognizing sensory awareness.

Tasks overview for Step 5

The tasks you will engage in during Step 5 are:

- Use the checklist to see how you are doing.

- Play games for at least ten minutes each day.

- Keep diaries for positives and difficult times.

- Find teachable moments.

Parent's checklist – self-monitoring

Before we discuss the skills for Step 5 we introduce a way for you to review those skills you have already learnt in previous steps – a short questionnaire based on the skills we have discussed so far in the programme. By completing this you will be able to see how you are doing in using the ideas we have given you in this self-help book. Are there some skills and tasks you find easier to do than others? We all tend to avoid doing what we find difficult. Or we may just have forgotten to do some stages in the programme. The questionnaire is a way for you to check for yourself which things you are doing well, and what needs further practice. It is sometimes helpful to complete this with your partner as you will each have things that you find easier to do and you may be able to support one another with ideas you find difficult. This is a guide to help you reflect on what you have learned over the last four steps and to provide you with the chance to see how things are going. Take some time to complete it and think about what it shows. Making changes in your parenting is hard, as is changing your child's behaviour, but the questionnaire will show you how much you have achieved already.

Parent's checklist

	Not at all	A little	Often
1. I remember to get my child's attention before giving instructions.			
2. I remember to use eye contact.			
3. I am good at giving praise.			
4. My partner and I work closely together to manage our child.			
5. I am consistent.			
6. I give clear messages to my child.			
7. I use countdowns when my child needs to change from what they are doing.			
8. I have clear behaviour boundaries.			
9. I avoid rows and keep calm.			
10. I practise giving my child limited choices.			
11. I use the word 'we' rather than 'you'.			
12. I play for at least ten minutes each day with my child.			
13. I have practised using quiet time with my child.			
14. I make sure I speak with the appropriate voice to my child.			
15. I talk about how I feel and encourage my child to do the same.			
16. I listen to what my child is saying to me.			
17. I try to expand his play by describing what he is doing.			
18. I manage any outbursts well.			
19. I manage to anticipate and distract my child preventing most outbursts.			
20. I use timers often.			
21. I praise my child's behaviour to others (Granny etc).			
22. I remember to repeat instructions to my child.			
23. I have clearly displayed house rules.			
24. I regularly review my child's ability in order to help them progress.			
25. I regularly reflect on how I am doing as a parent.			

Skill 1: Listening, sharing feelings, mutual respect and negotiations

Learning how to talk with children is perhaps the most important part of child-rearing. It will be how your child learns to talk with others and therefore how they behave outside the home. All children are born with their own individual personalities. At the same time many environmental factors influence the way a child behaves. The main factors are how you as their parent:

- guide and advise your child

- nurture your child

- establish rules and boundaries, setting limits

- protect your child's feelings and manage their influence on their self-esteem and social skills

- negotiate with your child.

All of the above are carried out through communication and by example. The statement 'They will grow out of it!' is often an excuse. Unacceptable behaviour that is not helped will only get worse. It is difficult to control young children, however if behaviour is not checked it will be worse when they are older, because the foundations of good communication and boundaries have not been established.

Talking helps to develop language skills and children's ability to express themselves and communicate with other people. Listening to your child develops in your child a sense of being understood and respected. This will help your child feel acknowledged and trusted. It will also make them feel safe. They need to feel safe enough to be able to tell you when life gets difficult for them, however hard or awful what they recount may be for you to listen to as a parent. It is at these times that they need to trust you to help them, even if they realize you may also be cross with them. Learning the skill of listening and paying attention, acknowledging different viewpoints to your child as a parent, is an art too.

Many families find it very difficult to express in words how they feel. If this is hard for the adult, it is near impossible for the child. Many children who have difficulties with their emotions struggle because they do not know the words to describe and make sense of what they are feeling. Your child needs examples, and they need to hear the right words used to describe emotions. They need to know how to explore emotions using words and ideas pitched at the appropriate developmental stage for them. It will help if you can use emotion words in your everyday language (e.g. 'I feel cross because I can't open this jar').

Apologize – it is healthy to apologize. If you apologize, your child will learn to say sorry too. It is important to make it clear what you are apologizing for. Ensure that you mean what you say and that your voice tone matches what you are saying. The way you use language with your child at home has a direct and immediate effect on how they will interact with other people outside the home.

Skill 2: Extending the use of timers

We talked about using timers in the first two steps to help your child learn about the concept of time and to put boundaries around activities.

Timers can be useful for a number of reasons.

- They can help your child learn to wait for something, for example a parent might say when the timer goes off then you can have… (see coping with delay in earlier steps).

- They can help them play for longer and build up their concentration: 'How long do you think you can play with the jigsaw today?'

- They can help your child by providing them with a boundary. They give a start and an ending which is visible: 'See if you can get dressed by the time the timer goes off.'

- They can be used to help your child set their own time, for example a parent may say 'You know you will have to wait to do that, how long do you think you can wait today?' This helps your child to think about their waiting time and they can be encouraged to increase how long they can wait.

- They give your child the seeds of the understanding of time perception and how long it takes to do things. Remember some children with ADHD have problems with this. So 'Let's see how long you are in the shower today' or 'You need to brush your teeth for at least two minutes; let's see how long you brush them for today.'

Using the timer can help your child start to learn to regulate themselves and understand their own difficulties, as well as providing them with the skills to manage them.

Skill 3: Calming your child outside the home

We have talked about keeping calm and speaking respectfully to your child and what to do when things are difficult. These are all good techniques to help your child. Children with ADHD tend to be 'always on the go'. Your child may find it hard to relax and sit still for any length of time. To help your child with this there are some ideas below. Each child is different and relaxation skills can take time to learn, so you may need to practise with your child for a while before they get the hang of them.

TIPS ON HELPING YOUR CHILD TO RELAX

- ▶ Have a designated quiet time during the day when your child listens to relaxing music or reads quietly.

- ▶ Some children like to soak in a warm bath with bubbles.

- ▶ Some children like to have their feet massaged.

- ▶ Some children like to have their back tickled.

- ▶ Lying quietly on the floor while you tell each other stories can be relaxing – as long as the stories are relaxing too!

- ▶ Some children find using mindfulness exercises relaxing.

Children with ADHD are good at being active, but they need to learn that not everyone can keep up with them.

Try to identify the activities that most suit your child which they can do to relax. It may be watching TV, having a massage or listening to music. This is an important skill for them to learn as they often have a great deal of energy, so they can exhaust themselves and others!

Helping your child relax will help them with friendships and relationships in later life. If your child learns to relax properly at home they will be calmer outside the home too.

Planning trips out

It is important to remember that your child needs to know the plan for the day.

If you are planning to go to the supermarket and you know that this can sometimes cause your child to get bored and become cross, then remind them that you must go shopping. You will be as quick as you can. They can help by getting some of the things for you. If they can be helpful and not get cross then they will have a reward (which you have agreed on before you go). Remember supermarkets are noisy and distracting for young children and your child may find it difficult to go there. Make the trip as short as possible and encourage good behaviour by keeping them involved.

Try to anticipate when your child is getting cross, then try to distract them and encourage them to sit quietly. If they do have a meltdown, take them off to one side and, if distraction does not work, sit with them and ignore them, keeping them safe until they stop. If this does not work, abandon the shopping and take them out of the shop. Find a calm place and wait – if you have a car you can return to it.

The most important factors are:

- planning the outing carefully for a time when you and they are not tired

- making it as short as possible initially – you can increase the time once you have scoped how long they can manage

- keeping them involved and interested so they do not become bored

- praising good behaviour

- giving a reward at the end (remember, a small reward, maybe one you have already agreed on).

Skill 4: Doing more on earshotting – showing others your child's good points

Previously mentioned in Step 2, this is the simple technique of talking about the positive behaviour your child has demonstrated, when they can hear you – to partners, friends or relatives. It is a good way of raising your child's self-esteem while encouraging others to see the good in your child. Children with ADHD are often seen as naughty by other people and this is a good way of ensuring their good points are seen too. Remember to keep doing this when you are outside the home and have the opportunity. It is important for your child to know you think highly of them.

Skill 5: Repetition of instructions

Getting your child to repeat instructions is a good way of reminding them of the task in hand and helping them with their memory. Remember children with ADHD have short-term memory problems. This means your child can often remember what happened months ago but not what you just asked them to do. If your child seems to have difficulty with this a good way to help them is to ask them gently to tell you what they must do, for example 'Is it time to put your shoes on?' Then ask the child 'What did Mummy/Daddy just ask you to do?' Remember instructions should be short. Give no more than one or two instructions at a time. Do not ask your child to repeat what you asked them to do every time, just occasionally and when it is important for your child to remember something. Remember having ADHD is exhausting for the child, trying to recollect everything people are saying is so hard for them – *be their 'safe' place someone who knows and understands them.*

Skill 6: Using house rules in the outside world

As we have seen, house rules can be very helpful in several ways. They can give you a chance to think about what is really important for your family to stick to. They also give you a chance to discuss with others who live in the household what is important to them, so that you can find a way of working together and discussing issues that affect you all. House rules need to be kept by everyone and (if possible) by visitors to your home. It is helpful as far as possible to have the same rules at Granny's, your childminder's and other places your child visits outside the home too.

Rules should be simple, with consequences if they are broken. This means that the results of breaking a rule should be thought out in advance with an appropriate sanction agreed. As with any sanction or consequence, this should be for a short duration and repeatable if necessary. Sanctions ideally should be agreed by everyone in advance, including the children.

Here are some examples which parents have used as house rules with appropriate sanctions: swearing or hitting little brother – sanction is that the child loses half an hour of TV time. For jumping on the furniture the sanction is having to sit quietly for two or three minutes.

Sanctions that are short can easily be repeated and therefore can have more impact than longer ones, when the child with ADHD has forgotten what the sanction was applied for. Remember the sanction should be fair and understandable. You can see above that hitting resulted in a longer and more serious sanction than jumping on the furniture. It is important to make that clear to the child, because if they are sent to their room for the same length of time whatever they do, the consequence will not have the same value.

Having established agreed house rules is a good way of applying rules without appearing to nag. Parents can say 'Oh dear, I see you have broken the rule and that means you must do... Never mind, I am sure you will remember that rule soon.' As your child grows older you can ask if there is anything you can do to help them remember the rule. This way you are encouraging your child to take responsibility for their behaviour and to see that they can learn, with help, to remember the rules themselves. It is good preparation for school when often classroom rules are set out at the beginning of each school year. Even children with ADHD will quickly know the school rules because they are clearly stated and are usually displayed on the wall. Giving the children a visual reminder helps.

It is worth remembering that sanctions alone are not a good method of ensuring your child behaves. There has to be a balance between rewards for good behaviour and sanctions. Praise works much better that sanctions in the long run, as it teaches your child how you want them to behave, not how you don't want them to! If possible, move to agreeing positive rules such as: we walk slowly, speak to each other respectfully (nicely), and praise your child for keeping these rules. *The better established the rules are at home, the more your child and you will naturally apply them when outside the home.*

TIPS ON HOUSE RULES

It is important that you work together on boundaries, limits and rewards. Work with your partner and child to set boundaries and discuss what will happen if these are broken.

Be consistent, fair, but firm, about enforcing sanctions if rules are broken.

Help your child to remember the rules and make sure they understand the consequences of breaking them.

Remind your child if you see that they are about to break a rule, to give them the opportunity to change their own behaviour.

It does not need two parents to enforce a sanction. Both parents individually should be able to enforce a sanction when needed. The parent who is not enforcing the sanction can help the child to act differently next time by saying something like 'It was a shame Mum had to give you that sanction. I wonder what you could do differently next time to avoid this?' Get the child to come up with ideas. That way they may learn different ways of acting. It is important that you give your child time to calm down before doing this. They need to be able to come up with ideas with your help.

Remember to use rewards as well as sanctions as much as possible to raise your child's self-esteem.

Skill 7: Using rewards

Children generally respond better to rewards than to sanctions and children with ADHD are no different in this respect, except that they are often told off for behaviour that is part of their nature. For example, they might be reprimanded for fidgeting or shouting out rather than putting their hand up in class. These difficulties arise because of your child's ADHD characteristics. They are something they can only learn to modify with time and with your support.

Rewards are therefore very important to raise your child's self-esteem about things that they can do well. Rewards should be inexpensive. They can include spending quality time with your child, for example going to the park after school, playing a game together or making up stories. You could give your child tokens to collect. For example, when they have five tokens that would equal a trip to the park. If you use tokens, make sure you do not take them away once the child has earned them. Apply a different sanction instead. As well as rewarding specific tasks remember to reward when your child is not expecting it and you see them do something well.

Skill 8: Using teachable moments in depth

Remember to practise the skills your child is learning outside the home. The good work you are doing with your child at home will help enormously when you are out, and teachable moments not only extend your child's learning but also show them that the changes you are making in your parenting and communication styles apply as much outside in public as they do back home.

For example, counting games can be done walking along the road. Matching the same type of car or lorry can be a good way of making sure your child pays attention. Supermarkets are great learning places as long as you're not doing the weekly shop – choose a time when you are not rushed. Get your child to collect two tins of beans that look the same, for example. Or you could take the labels with you and ask your child to find the tins or packets that match what they have on their list. At the checkout see if you can distract them while they wait and remember to praise them for waiting. Practising will help your child learn by reinforcement (doing things over and over till they get the hang of it).

As we have seen, magic carpets can easily be transported to Granny's or the shop if necessary. As we discussed earlier you could keep a square of carpet or a scarf in your bag that could be used as the transportable 'calming down square'.

Skill 9: Using Social Stories

Social Stories are very useful for children who have difficulty in understanding social situations. So they are worth trying if your child finds some social situations difficult. They are written is a specific way and this is important. How to write the stories is outlined below. We have included an example for you too.

While Social Stories are not directly used to alter behaviour they are useful to help children understand why they are being asked not to do something. They explain the effects their behaviour has on other people and themselves and so are particularly useful if your child has problems seeing things from others' viewpoints.

A Social Story is a short story written especially for your child to help them understand a particular social situation that they find challenging or confusing (e.g. dinner time, bath time, bed time, play time with a brother or sister) and help them know what behaviour is expected of them.

The story describes the situation and includes details of where and when the activity will take place, what will happen, how other people may be feeling (e.g. Emily feels sad when I take her teddy away from her) and why the child should behave in a certain way (e.g. Mummy will be really pleased when I eat my carrots).

Social Stories also include lots of pictures. These can be actual photographs of your child acting out the story. They can also include themes and characters that your child is especially interested in, to help increase their level of interest and motivation towards reading the story.

Writing a Social Story

Step 1: Picture the goal

What do you want your child to be able to understand/achieve? (e.g. eat his dinner without starting a fight with his sister)

Step 2: Gather information

When and where does the situation occur?

Who is involved?

What happens? (set out what you would like the child to do, step-by-step)

How will other people be feeling?

Step 3: Tailor the text

Make sure the story fits with the interests and abilities of your child. Photos or pictures can be added. There are some ready-made stories available (e.g. C. Gray (2000) *The New Social Story Book: Illustrated Edition*) and these can be a helpful starting point. There are stories on a range of topics, such as sharing, going to the hairdressers etc.

It is very important to include a sentence on how pleased you will be when your child behaves the way you would like them to and include details of any reward they might get for doing as they are told.

Social Stories are good because they:

- are visual

- provide a clear message

- are permanent

- are individual for your specific child

- are practical

- provide an opportunity for children to practise skills before attempting the real situation.

How to use Social Stories

Try reading the story once a day – immediately before the situation in question if possible (e.g. just before lunch time, if this is what the story is about).

You will need to review the story and how your child is getting on after about a week or two. Do you think it is working? How will you know if it is working or not?

If it has not been working, do you have the right focus for the story? How could it be changed/improved?

How will you celebrate your child's achievement?

The role of a Social Story is to explain and demonstrate in a story the way a person should act or behave. These are particularly useful if your child has any neurodivergence, such as autism. What they do is describe a situation in detail to the child.

Skill 10: Using mindfulness

There have been some studies looking at mindfulness in treating adults and children who have ADHD. Mindfulness is a way of being in the here and now with your child – so that you concentrate on the time you are spending in the present rather than worrying about the past or the future. Some parents and children find this approach helpful in focusing on what is important to them now. They can find it helps them to relax. It is not a relaxation method but a way of noticing your thoughts and how these can influence your behaviour. It is also a way of becoming more aware of them.

Patterns of behaviour are often automatic, and it is not until we become aware of them that we are able to see if they are helpful or not. So these exercises are designed to give you a brief introduction to mindfulness to see if you as a parent find it helpful in raising your awareness. The exercise for your child focuses on their senses and hopefully will help them become more aware of these (smell, taste, hearing, touch and sight) as a way of slowing down and noticing things more. Later in the book we will give you some mindfulness exercises to do with your child.

There are many free mindfulness exercises that can be downloaded from the web, for example: www.bbcchildreninneed.co.uk/schools/primary-school/mindfulness-hub.

Skill 11: Using a sensory tool kit

Building on from the mindfulness for children where they become more aware of their senses, this sensory tool kit provides you as parents with ideas to help your child. Many children with ADHD have different sensory profiles, some may react intensively to smells and if you wear a certain perfume you might notice their behaviour worsening. Some react to sounds – you might see your child appear in distress at fireworks or loud sirens. As parents in our busy everyday lives it can be difficult to notice sensory responses.

Tasks for Step 5

Use the checklist at the beginning of this step to see how you are doing. Note the things you find the easiest to do and those you find more difficult. Discuss these with your partner or friend and seek their support if you wish.

Try to find teachable moments in everyday life, so that your use of the skills is transferred across all situations and places. The more you practise the more confident you become and the skills will become second nature to you.

Remember to keep playing with your child for ten minutes each day. Your child will respond to your consistency and over time will learn from this. Behaviour changes in children with ADHD take longer to appear but are very worthwhile.

Parents with symptoms of ADHD themselves

We mentioned at the beginning of the Six-Step Programme that parents with ADHD themselves may have more difficulty than parents without ADHD in carrying out the skills and tasks. We suggest that this is because of their own ADHD symptoms. *If you think your parenting is being affected by your ADHD symptoms, ask someone you trust to help you.* See if they can notice tasks or situations you find difficult and support you in doing these. It is important that you do not choose someone who will take over and direct your behaviour too much as this will only lessen your own self-esteem in managing your child. Pick someone who can help you over time, who understands ADHD and who you like! A sense of humour may help too.

Remember to keep up using the diaries.

Recap and review
Goal for Step 5
The goal for Step 5 was to review how you are getting on with the skills you have learned and to transfer these to situations outside the home.

Skills summary for Step 5
The skills you have practised are: (tick those you have used)

1. I am listening, sharing feelings, respecting and negotiating with my child.

2. I have been expanding the use of timers.

3. I have found ways of calming my child.

4. I have used 'earshotting' to others about my child.

5. I remember to repeat instructions to help my child to remember.

6. I have practised using house rules outside the home.

7. I reward my child.

8. I have found lots of teachable moments.

9. I have written a Social Story for my child.

10. I have practised mindfulness with my child.

11. I am noticing how my child is reacting to different senses.

Tasks summary for Step 5
The tasks you carried out were:

- I have used the checklist to see how I am doing.

- I've played games for at least ten minutes each day.

- I have been keeping diaries for positives and for difficult times.

- I have practised finding teachable moments.

Diary for good days

Day/Date . . . .

Time . . . .

What made it good? . . . .
. . . .
. . . .
. . . .

What did you do? [praise, smile, emoji] . . . .
. . . .
. . . .
. . . .

Did it help your child? . . . .
. . . .
. . . .
. . . .
. . . .

How do you feel now? . . . .
. . . .
. . . .
. . . .

How do you think your child feels now? . . . .
. . . .
. . . .
. . . .
. . . .

Diary for difficult days

Day/Date . . . .

Time . . . .

Trigger (what led up to the difficulty) . . . .
. . . .
. . . .

What happened? . . . .
. . . .
. . . .

What did you do? . . . .
. . . .
. . . .

Did it help? . . . .
. . . .
. . . .

How do you feel now? . . . .
. . . .
. . . .

How do you think your child feels now? . . . .
. . . .
. . . .

Looking back would you do anything different? . . . .
. . . .
. . . .

STEP 6

Times Ahead

GOAL FOR STEP 6
The goal of Step 6, the final stage in the programme, is for you to continue to transfer all the skills you have learnt in this book to everyday situations and to plan how to use them in the future, especially at times around transitions to new stages and places, such as when your child starts or changes school.

Skills overview for Step 6

The two important skills we focus on in this chapter are:

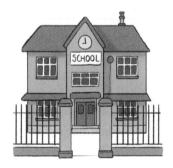

1. How to cope during difficult times.

2. How to seek help when you need it.

Tasks overview for Step 6

The tasks you practise in this final step are:

- Review the skills learned in previous steps.

- Remember to scope and reassess your child's abilities as they grow older.

- Remember to look after yourselves.

- Look at the scenarios in order to review the skills you have attained.

- Preparing your child for school or going from infants to juniors.

- Working together with schools.

Introduction to Step 6

This step is about preparing for the future. By now you will have been practising and gaining confidence in using the skills we have covered and seeing an improvement in how your child responds to you.

We know that children with ADHD have difficulties in times of transition, that is, in changing from one situation to another. This could be transitions between parents' homes if you are separated, or changing from infant to junior school, for example.

It is important that periods of transition are planned for and your child is prepared for being in different settings. This means working closely together and providing as much consistency as possible between the two places. In order to do this good communication is essential. If you are having difficulties achieving this, seek help from professional services early on.

Skill 1: How to cope during difficult times

There are always times in our lives when events challenge us. These include times of bereavement, loss, relationship difficulties or financial difficulty. At these times children pick up on the anxieties of the adults around them. Children's behaviour often appears worse around these times, and children with ADHD are no exception.

This can be for several reasons. It may be that you have reduced the amount of time you spend with your child, without realizing it, because of the difficulties. Your child with ADHD may react in several different ways. They might become angry – and this might feel like you are back to how it was before the programme and your interventions. They might demand more attention and not always in a positive way. If you have had a stressful time and your child's behaviour is worsening when it had been good before, it is worth reading the relevant pages of this book again to remind you of what you may have stopped doing. For example, sometimes parents relax the house rules unconsciously because of the difficulties they are going through, and this can lead to children acting out to check that the boundaries remain the same. *It is important that you re-establish rules and boundaries as soon as you feel able.* This will help to settle the child's behaviour again.

Children often blame themselves for things that happen. Your child might think 'Mum and Dad are in a bad mood because I wanted breakfast at the wrong moment,' when parents may have just had a disagreement. Or 'Granny died because I was naughty.' These events are obviously not the child's fault. Reassuring the child and talking about your feelings helps your child to understand why times are difficult.

Parental disagreement and arguments can be very upsetting for children. They generally love both their parents and need to be kept out of adult conflict.

Skill 2: Seeking help when you need it

If the situation is very difficult, and you are struggling to cope, seek support from people you trust. This could be a close friend or relative or a professional. Health visitors, school nurses or your doctor can advise you or point you in the direction of someone willing to and qualified to help. Don't be afraid to ask. Mediation can really help parents who are struggling to communicate.

Tasks for Step 6
Reflection on the previous steps and reassessing your older child

Continue with all the skills you have learned from Steps 1–5. We suggest that you continue to work on all of the suggestions from Step 1 through to 5. Eventually the approach will become second nature. The tips that you have learned work well with all children; you can use them with your other children also. Remember that this programme is for younger children, but the steps can be easily adapted as the child develops. *The same principles remain, you just have to adapt them to the age of your child.*

For example, *quiet time* for teenagers is often in their room, and choices would probably be around clothes or music, for example 'Do you want this music download or that one?', 'These trainers or those?', 'Do you want to do the dishes now or after *Eastenders*?'

Helping children and adolescents with their *time perception* would consist of day or weekly planners, getting them to estimate how long tasks take them to complete and then timing themselves to see if they can judge time.

Play and games would be around more sophisticated games such as 'sets' where they have to use visual skills by identifying shapes, colours and patterns. Family games are also useful as a way of helping your teenager learn to take turns, cope with losing and have fun. For example, Upwords, Catchphrase, Guess Who, Rummikub, Jenga and so forth.

Looking after yourselves

Children with ADHD can be hard work. The aim of this book has been to support you in becoming your child's guide and trainer to help them overcome some of their difficulties and help you feel confident in managing their behaviour.

Even with all the skills you may have been using already and with what new knowledge you may have acquired, parenting is still hard work. It is important that you *find ways of supporting yourself* in this vital parenting role. Many parents have told us how difficult it is to find time for themselves or indeed time to spend with their partner, if they are in a relationship. If you are in any doubt, *think about what your child is learning from you as their role model.* Being a role model for your child is not easy but by showing your child that you need time for you, or for you and your partner, you are demonstrating how you maintain your own well-being and relationships with others. So if they go on to having relationships as they grow older, they have learned from you how to keep relationships going.

Generalizing and extending

This is the last step of the programme – by now you should have been able to put into practice what you have learnt. It is important to realize though that change rarely occurs overnight and that it will often take a few months to see a significant improvement. *Changing your parenting approach can be difficult*: keep using the guidelines.

Forgive yourself if you cannot practise them all of the time, we are all human. Just try to achieve as much as is possible. We do know from other families that they work.

As already mentioned, this book can be used for all children, so if you have other children who are less hyperactive it can help them too. It is, however, specifically aimed at children with ADHD. We have found that for some parents it helps to use the book at least two or three times over a period of few months. You should keep going back through this self-help book until you are very familiar with all the ideas in it. Some parents will find some ideas easier to work with than others. It can be simple persistence with a particular approach that works in the end, so don't be disheartened if at first things don't appear to change, or if you get times when strategies work less well... Thinking about the long term: this programme can be used with children over longer periods of time if necessary.

The power of NFPP emojis

As part of looking after yourself we encourage you to ask other people to help make time for you. Remember it is important that you look after yourself, or else you won't be able to look after your child. So ask your partner and family members to create some space and time for you. It may be time for you to spend time with friends, get a haircut, find some time to go shopping alone (when you have time to try stuff on!) or just relax. While you are away you may get calls or text from home with messages about how difficult things are. Don't cut your plans short but do be supportive of whoever is looking after your child, you do know how challenging it can be.

Instead of making suggestions for how they can better manage your child in your absence, use emojis to remind them about NFPP strategies that they have read about in this book, and strategies you have no doubt already explained to them. Ideally, we would like you to create your own emojis for NFPP strategies but if you don't know how to do that, or frankly don't have the time, below are some suggestions from us for the key NFPP strategies.

So imagine you are mum of a 7-year-old boy with ADHD and a

4-year-old boy without ADHD, and you have finally managed to find time to meet a close friend for lunch, in a restaurant that doesn't give out balloons and free ice cream. Just as you pull into the car park, your partner texts to say he is having a really difficult time and can't get the 7-year-old to have lunch. Don't cancel your own lunch, just remind your partner: Perspex shield 🛡 Recruit attention 👥 Two choices 😠 Praise ✔ and they should be fine.

Suggested emojis for key NFPP strategies

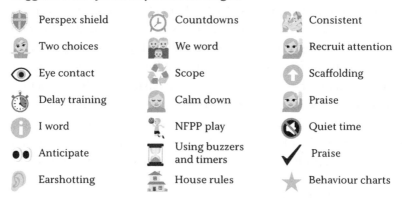

🛡	Perspex shield	⏰	Countdowns	👪	Consistent
😠	Two choices	👪	We word	👀	Recruit attention
👁	Eye contact	♻	Scope	⬆	Scaffolding
⏱	Delay training	😣	Calm down	😊	Praise
ⓘ	I word	🤾	NFPP play	🚫	Quiet time
●●	Anticipate	⏳	Using buzzers and timers	✔	Praise
👂	Earshotting	🏠	House rules	⭐	Behaviour charts

Communication with school – preparing your child for changing school

You might find that the times when your child changes from nursery to school, or from infants to juniors or from junior to senior school, throw up the most difficulties. If so, you may want to go back to study the guidance here again, as at times of developmental change your child may find life difficult and seem to regress. Having to sit still for long periods, coping with school rules, having to wait their turn, doing homework...all these are difficult and challenging skills for the child with ADHD.

You can prepare your child for changes in school. Their school will be doing that too. Parents should, if they are happy about doing so, let the child's school know that their child has ADHD and show the child's teacher this self-help book so they can think about whether any of the strategies in it would be helpful to the teaching staff.

TIPS ON EASING SCHOOL TRANSITION

- ► Help your child to sit still and do colouring or games or look at a book for increasing lengths of time, in preparation for school.

- ► Get your child to practise asking their sister, brother or their friends for toys without snatching.

- ► Make it clear to your child who will take them to school and pick them up.

Your child will not always remember what you have told them. They may get anxious, and if they are anxious they may appear cross with you or someone else. Sometimes leaving them a reminder note in their lunchbox may help them to recollect what is happening for the rest of the day. Notes of encouragement will help them feel reassured during the day.

To conclude: general hints and tips

Children with ADHD are hard to parent; they need a different sort of parenting in order for them to learn from you, they call on all your parenting skills. Continue to work with your partner to be consistent with the messages you present to your child.

Go back to the beginning of the book if you need to remind yourself what to do. Use the checklists to see if you are maintaining the use of the skills. *Be kind to yourself.* Seek the support of others to let off steam too. Make sure you have time to yourself and with your partner. It is a good example to set, as well as essential to maintain your relationship.

Forgive yourself if you have a bad day – we all do sometimes. Enlist the support of others. Family and friends can be lifesavers when the going gets tough.

We have included some scenarios for you to practise the skills you've acquired, and you can review how your interactions are going. You will find these in the Resources section at the back of the book.

We have put another copy of the parent's checklist in the Resources for you to remind yourself how you are doing, and to remind you to check up on tasks you may need to go back and revise. The numbers for the skills, the table of contents and the index should help you locate the areas of the book you want to return to.

Remember your child's symptoms should become easier for you and for them to control as time goes on with the programme, but school might be a challenge (which can be positive as well as negative).

Note about medication

While we know that the strategies given in this book help children with ADHD, we have not discussed the use of medication which can also help children with ADHD. Combining these strategies for some children may mean that a lower dose of medication and therefore fewer side effects can together bring about significant change for the child with ADHD, especially in school. Further information would be available from your primary care doctor, clinic doctor or nurse. You may well not need further help but, if you do, try to see professionals in a favourable light. They can help.

By reading this book and adopting the strategies suggested you are well on the way to improving things for you, your child and your family. Congratulations and very best wishes for the future.

Diary for good days

Day/Date . . . .

Time . . . .

What made it good? . . . .
. . . .
. . . .
. . . .

What did you do? [praise, smile, emoji] . . . .
. . . .
. . . .
. . . .

Did it help your child? . . . .
. . . .
. . . .
. . . .
. . . .

How do you feel now? . . . .
. . . .
. . . .
. . . .

How do you think your child feels now? . . . .
. . . .
. . . .
. . . .
. . . .

Diary for difficult days

Day/Date . . . .

Time . . . .

Trigger (what led up to the difficulty) . . . .
. . . .
. . . .

What happened? . . . .
. . . .
. . . .

What did you do? . . . .
. . . .
. . . .

Did it help? . . . .
. . . .
. . . .

How do you feel now? . . . .
. . . .
. . . .

How do you think your child feels now? . . . .
. . . .
. . . .

Looking back would you do anything different? . . . .
. . . .
. . . .

Resources

The scenarios below are fictional but draw on our extensive experience of working with children with ADHD and their parents. You should treat them as multiple-choice quizzes.

Practice scenarios

Tom is always having problems playing; his concentration is poor, lasting only a few minutes. What can you do?

1. Tell him he has to sit down and play.

2. Ignore this, he will learn one day.

3. Help him by setting regular time aside to play with him to enable him to practise.

Clue: Children with ADHD often miss vital steps in how to play.

* * *

You sent Rachael upstairs to get her school bag. She hasn't returned downstairs and she will be late for school. Do you:

1. Remind Rachael what she went for and give her a time limit to come downstairs with it?

2. Shout at Rachael; tell her she will be late?

3. Go upstairs and get the bag yourself?

Clue: Children with ADHD have short-term memory problems.

* * *

Jimmy comes out of school and runs about dangerously all the way home. Do you:

1. Pick him up in the car?

2. Put him on reins to ensure he is embarrassed in front of his friends and will stop running about?

3. Understand that he probably needs to be active after a day concentrating; arrange a deal that if he walks next to you he can go to the park on the way home?

Clue: ADHD children find it hard to concentrate all day; they need to let off steam.

* * *

Bradley's teacher meets you when you pick him up asking to have a word about their difficult behaviour, you talk to her. Do you:

1. Feel embarrassed, tell Bradley off on the way home – ask him why he is so naughty?

2. Wait until you get home, talk to Bradley about his day, what was good and what wasn't, and give him ideas to prevent it happening again.

3. Punish him when you get home – it is important to make sure he knows he will be punished if he is naughty again.

Clue: Children with ADHD find it hard to problem solve. By exploring difficulties freely, you can help them learn to act differently.

* * *

Bradley is still having difficulties in school; the teacher calls you in for the third time that week. Do you:

1. Go in and speak to him, feel embarrassed and helpless and go home?

2. Ask a friend/partner to join you, arrange a further regular time to meet and ask the teacher what support is being arranged for Bradley and himself in school?

3. Stop picking him up from school, send a friend?

Clue: It is important that you obtain as much support for your child and possible and that people coming into contact with him understand his difficulties.

* * *

You tell Amy off. She shouts and says you don't love her. Do you:

- Tell her you don't love her?

- Get upset, plead with her that you do?

- Say to her that you think she is upset that you have told her off, that you do love her but that she has to stop what she is doing.

Clue: Be strong. Separate the behaviour from the child, while being consistent.

Mindfulness exercises with your child
Eating mindfully

You might want to practise the stages alongside your child so that you build your experiences together. There are no right or wrong answers — this is an exercise that brings your attention into the present.

During the exercise it doesn't matter what your feelings and thoughts are or what your child's are. It's OK, there is no need to judge these. Just accept them. All thoughts and feelings are OK whether they are positive or negative – they are just thoughts coming and going.

It is worth preparing your child by telling them that they have to wait a very short while before you start the exercise together and that you will be looking at a piece of apple very carefully before you eat it together. Taking an apple, cut two slices and put these to the side. Take hold of the rest of the apple.

Spend time looking at the apple. What do you see? Notice its colour. Are there differences in its colour – does it change? What does your child notice about the colours? Don't ask them to name the colours correctly: this exercise is to help them look at patterns and shading rather than colours. You want them to really explore the apple and to give it their full attention.

Ask them if they can see where it was joined to the tree. Is the stalk still present? Has it any leaves on it? Take a moment to think together out loud about the tree it came from: wonder if it had lots of leaves, think about the blossom that turned into this apple, the bees that helped pollinate the blossom; now think about the trunk of the tree and the roots deep into the ground drawing up all the nutrients to the tree to help grow this apple. Imagine the tree swaying in the breeze with the apple growing on it; the wind and rain and sunshine that it will have experienced before it left the tree. Think about it separating from the tree and starting its journey with the support of the grower – perhaps how carefully the grower had prepared the apple for its journey, maybe by carefully placing it with other apples to start the journey. It may have been wrapped to prevent bruising on its travels from the grower to the lorry. Think together about the journey with other apples to the supermarket, the towns and villages it may have passed through on its journey to your hand.

Now take one slice in your hand and put the other in your child's hand. Touch it and ask them to touch it with their fingers. Does it feel rough or smooth? Hot or cold? Wet or dry? What else do they notice? What else do you notice? Talk about what you have both noticed. It's OK for your child not to say anything — the prompts are for you to talk about with your child to increase their attention.

Encourage your child to put it to his ear. Can they hear anything? If they shake it does it make any noise – if they dig their fingers in, it may. Can you hear anything? They may find this funny, and that is OK. Again, talk about what you have noticed as well.

Now smell it. What can they smell? You may need to help them with words – is it a strong smell or just a slight smell? Sweet or savoury? Notice whether this is pleasant or unpleasant. Notice if either of you is making any judgements about the apple.

Acknowledge these, and see if it is possible to let go of these and just experience it as it is.

Each of you bring the apple to your mouth, noticing any movement in your muscles contracting and expanding, and noticing readiness in your mouth. Bring it to your lips, touch it with your lips, now lick it. What does your child notice in their mouth? Is it watering? Does it feel comfortable, do they want to eat more? What is its texture like to their tongue — rough or smooth? Notice any judgements about its taste.

Now take a bite and chew it. Is it noisy now, what can they hear? What can they taste? What do you hear and taste? Is your child chewing slowly or fast? Are you chewing slowly or fast? What do you notice about your mouth - is it watering more or less? What is it like when you swallow? Lumpy or smooth, comfortable or not? What do your teeth feel?

What feelings are you both left with? Wanting more? Liking it? It doesn't matter - whatever their feelings and thoughts are it is OK. Whatever your feelings and thoughts are it is OK. There's no need to judge your thoughts or your child's - just accept them. All thoughts and feelings are OK, whether they are positive or negative — they are just thoughts and feelings coming and going.

Talk this exercise over with your child. Ask them what they noticed, and whether they liked doing it.

Applying hand cream

Choose a time when you need to help your child sit quietly. This could be during 'Quiet time' to allow time to be together. It might have the added benefit of helping them to calm down and sit for a while.

Tell them you are going to spend time together massaging their hand, and they in turn will massage yours.

Use some hand cream that you know they are not allergic to (you may have to try a small bit the day before to check for any allergies).

Spend a few moments thinking about the cream you are applying - the fragrance and where this came from, link to a plant that is growing (for example lavender), how this grows from seeds, gradually getting bigger and bigger until it blossoms. Think about the nutrients it receives from the ground and the gentle pruning and guidance it needs until it blossoms. Think together how the blossom looks – perhaps it appears confident and upright, swaying gently in the sun. Think about the purpose of the blossoms and how they may be collected to make the perfume to add to the cream to make it smell lovely and relaxing.

Notice together any thoughts or feelings you have about the cream. There is no need to judge these thoughts, notice them coming and going

Now get them to pay attention to their hands. Get them to really look at them. Are they rough or smooth, big or small, hot or cold? What do they notice on them? Are they clean or dirty? Do they have short or long nails? Are there any stains from food on them?

Then you look at their hands too. Make positive comments about them, for example 'They are lovely and soft hands; haven't you washed them well today' (if they are clean). Become aware of any other thoughts and judgements. Just let them come and go.

Then get them to look at your hands and to notice the same things – are they rough or smooth, big or small, hot or cold? Are they clean or dirty? Do you have short or long nails? Have they got any nail polish on them? Are there any stains from food on them?

Don't worry if they just listen to you asking these things, they do not need to answer.

Put a small dot of hand cream on their hand. Ask them to smell it: what can they smell? (You may need to help them with words.) Is it a strong smell or just a slight smell, sweet or savoury. Notice if they think it is pleasant or unpleasant. Do they like it? Do you like it? It's OK if you don't.

Massage their hands gently, noticing the texture, the temperature, the feel of each finger.

See what they notice about the hand massage. Gently encourage them to express what they notice – this could be anything. Listen to what they are saying. There is no need to reply to what they notice other than acknowledging what they say.

Tell them what you noticed.

Help them to massage your hands. Ask them what they notice, feel, smell and so on.

While doing this exercise your role is to bring your child's attention to the senses. It is not necessary for them to answer questions at the time. But once the massage has finished talk about it and what their thoughts and feelings were. There are no right or wrong thoughts for you or your child. These are your thoughts and feelings, simply how it is right now.

Review sheet

Use the review sheet below according to the instructions in Step 3: Helping Your Child's Attention and Concentration through Play. It is a very helpful tool for assessing your child's abilities. Make more of your own if you run out of space.

Review sheet

Date	
What are you observing?	
How long did it take your child to complete this task?	
Did your child manage these?	
Did they require help?	

Parent's checklist for self-monitoring

Here is a short questionnaire based on the ideas in the Six-Step Parenting Programme. We hope by completing this you can see how you are doing in using the tasks and skills we have introduced in the programme. Are there some you find easier to do than others? Sometimes we avoid doing what we find most difficult. Or we have just forgotten to do some tasks. The questionnaire is a way for you to check for yourself, and assess which strategies you are using well and what needs further practice. It is sometimes helpful to complete this with your partner, as you will each have things that you find easier to do and you may be able to support one another with aspects of the programme you find difficult.

Parent's checklist

	Not at all	A little	Often
1. I remember to get my child's attention before giving instructions.			
2. I remember to use eye contact.			
3. I am good at giving praise.			
4. My partner and I work closely together to manage our child.			
5. I am consistent.			
6. I give clear messages to my child.			
7. I use countdowns when my child needs to change from what they are doing.			
8. I have clear behaviour boundaries.			
9. I avoid rows and keep calm.			
10. I practise giving my child limited choices.			
11. I use the word 'we' rather than 'you'.			
12. I play for at least ten minutes each day with my child.			
13. I have practised using quiet time with my child.			
14. I make sure I speak with the appropriate voice to my child.			
15. I talk about how I feel and encourage my child to do the same.			
16. I listen to what my child is saying to me.			
17. I try to expand his play by describing what he is doing.			
18. I manage any outbursts well.			
19. I manage to anticipate and distract my child preventing most outbursts.			
20. I use timers often.			
21. I praise my child's behaviour to others (Granny etc).			
22. I remember to repeat instructions to my child.			
23. I have clearly displayed house rules.			
24. I regularly review my child's ability in order to help them progress.			
25. I regularly reflect on how I am doing as a parent.			

A final word

For some children parenting strategies will be sufficient, but for others it may be necessary to go on to consider medication. Generally speaking, guidance for doctors in the UK would not recommend medication for children with ADHD under 6 years of age. This may be different in other countries. Under 6 years of age in the UK, some prescribing practitioners will prescribe dexamphetamine or methylphenidate for children with severe difficulties if this seems warranted, however it is out of its licensed use and so it is important for parents to be aware of this and to discuss this with their clinician. Should medication need to be considered, a medical history should be taken to look for other possible reasons for the child having ADHD difficulties and also for possible medical contraindications to starting medication. Baseline monitoring should also be performed.

Index